# Do

The Complete Guide on How To Prepare a Homemade Delicacies for Dog to Live Healthy and Happy

CARLA WATERS

The information herein is offered for informational purposes solely, and is universal as so. The presentation of the information is without contract or any type of guarantee assurance.

The trademarks that are used are without any consent, and the publication of the trademark is without permission or backing by the trademark owner. All trademarks and brands within this book are for clarifying purposes only and are the owned by the owners themselves, not affiliated with this document.

# INTRODUCTION

It is possible to take care of pets economically and healthily. There are routines of buying food and the recipe for making homemade food. And this will encourage and help you make healthy and cheap meals for your Dog.

It is important not to confuse the recipe with leftover food. Human food can contain many spices that are a danger to the dog friend. According to veterinarians and nutritionists, onions, chocolate, and star fruit are prohibited foods. Garlic can be used to lower cholesterol and control hypertension.

Whether you want to try feeding your raw dog food or are looking for ideas for homemade dog food, the components of a good home dog food plan are not complicated, but they require diligence and dedication to you.

The calcium level in your Dog's diet is essential: you can't feed too much or too much. It is also necessary to balance the nutrients over time: mix and match different vegetables and meat over the weeks and years. So how do you ensure that your Dog's diet is complete and balanced? Great food should be ingested.

Three basic ingredients for homemade dog food:

1. Muscle

2. Bones and raw meat products (animal organs)

3. Vegetables (leafy, not starchy)

Whole Dog Journal avoids giving dog owners step-by-step recipes for raw or cooked dog food. We can share personal protocols of experienced companions with dogs to feed their home-prepared dogs. Still, you will soon realize that there is no perfect recipe for dog food and that your Dog gets all the necessary nutrients, you need many recipes that include many different ingredients of whole foods.

1. Meat muscle

We all know what it is. Chicken, lamb, beef, pork, deer, rabbit: these are the meat you see on commercial pet food labels and the type of meat people eat the most. Fish also fall into this food category: common fish meat that dogs eat includes mackerel and salmon. Unlike humans, there is no limit to the amount of protein a dog should eat; dogs can fully survive on animal meat if needed. It does not matter if the dogs eat raw meat, even if there have been cases where the dogs have been given salmonella or E. coli. Coli, it is rare and mostly comes down to a pre-existing lack of immunity.

2. Raw meat bones and other parts of animals

Here are the most complicated components of homemade dog food. Raw meat bones refer to a specific type of animal bone used for eating, not just chewing (we call them recreation bones). RMBs feed on untreated dogs, with muscles and tendons still tied. Therefore, they are not dried and are not brittle and are usually large enough not to be swallowed whole. Raw meat bones are an essential source of calcium for dogs; if for any reason, your Dog cannot tolerate RMB, alternatives such as ground bones or ground eggshells can provide calcium in their food.

Organic meats such as liver, kidneys, heart, and neck are also needed for dogs that are fed at home. In dogs fed raw foods, the organs should make up about 10% of the total diet, which can be a challenge for some dog keepers. Cow meat contains all the rich vitamins and minerals that make your dog shine, but since it is not widely consumed (at least in the United States), it is not widely available.

3. Vegetables

Which vegetables should you include in your Dog's diet? Many vegetables are good for dogs.

Spinach

Dear

pea

Lattuga

All kinds of zucchini (zucchini, zucchini, acorn, butter)

Cavolfiore

Broccoli

Cucumbers

Asparagus

Vegetables and fruit for the benefit of dogs, but not essential

sweet potatoes

celery

Cavolo

Cavolo

broccoli

tomato

mushrooms

Green beans (when cooked)

Any edible berries

Any type of melon

avocado

Mele

Orange

Pear Orange

Banana

Pineapple

Lemon and lime

There are plenty of plant-based nutritional options for dogs, but there are a handful of foods that dogs should avoid or limit consumption:

Cipolle

Aglio

Night Shadows (potatoes, eggplant, peppers)

Grapes and raisins

Does this food kill all the dogs that swallow them? Of course not. Some dogs eat potatoes and peppers all their lives and have no problems. Other dogs occasionally receive grapes as a gift, and they do well. Garlic in small amounts is good for dogs. The problem is that each of these ingredients contains toxins that, if consumed in excess, can cheer up your Dog, so it is not recommended to use it in homemade dog food.

**Cereals in Homemade Dog Food**

Dogs should not eat grains for a complete and balanced diet, nor should they eat beans and legumes. Cereals and beans are not bad for dogs; they are not just an important part of a dog's diet. As a source of protein, these starchy ingredients can be included in your Dog's meals from time to time, but they should not be the main ingredients in the home diet you plan.

When feeding our dogs, like cats, with the same dry food always raises questions about us, whether they are fed well enough, and more importantly, whether they are satisfied with this situation. In addition to refreshing ourselves, making foods with rich content at home will also appeal to our dogs' taste.

The following recipes are highly nutritious and healthy alternatives for dogs. We also have treats and chew food recipes. You can feed your homemade dog food if he does not have any health problems or conditions that require a special diet. On the other hand, there are some vitamins in dry foods that we cannot easily obtain.

# CHAPTER 1: DOG NUTRITION

## Personal theories about dog nutrition

Many myths revolve around the right dog nutrition. Some sound logical; others are difficult to understand. However, through the influence of dog food manufacturers and convenience, most dog owners have developed their theory on the subject. After all, you know your animal best! As far as certain preferences are concerned, that is correct. In other areas, it is worth listening to the advice of experts. Free from economic interests, the following ten rules apply to healthy and normal developed animals.

## The basics of dog nutrition

To understand the rules for correct dog nutrition and to implement them consistently, you should keep the parentage of your favorite in the back of your mind. As a direct descendant of wolves, he only differs genetically by 0.2% from his ancestors. The wolf feeds almost exclusively on unprocessed meat and only eats vegetable food if necessary. Therefore, the teeth are geared towards tearing and dividing; for example it is not suitable for grinding grain. The same applies to the domesticated house dog!

## BARF as a method of feeding dogs

Due to the convenience of the owners, over time, one switched to ready-made food. In order to increase the economic efficiency of the dog food, more and more vegetable ingredients were mixed in with it. Although this has a positive effect on the manufacturers' profits, it does not benefit the dogs. Barfen was created as a counterpoint to this (also BARFcalled: Biologically appropriate raw feeding). This movement is based on a fundamental attitude towards nutrition, similar to that of clean eaters or vegetarians. However, Barfer advocate feeding only fresh, unprocessed meat. Behind this is the pursuit of a natural diet that corresponds to the type of animal. Other carnivores, such as cats, are also fed this way. The main arguments for this are:

Knowledge of all components

Chewing instinct is better satisfied

Lower risk of dog food allergies

Counteracting health problems (gastrointestinal problems, skin diseases, kidney, and urinary tract infections, etc.)

Against dog nutrition with BARF

Of course, this calls for the large dog food corporations, which triggered this movement in the first place due to their lack of transparency in the processing and the increasing proportion of plant-based additives. But there are also some veterinarians among the opponents of the theory. They make the English meaning of barf advantage, which means to be sick means. The following concerns are cited:

Risk of malnutrition due to lack of nutrients

detailed knowledge of feed science is required for the compilation

incorrect use can trigger health problems (gastrointestinal problems, diarrhea, constipation, broken teeth, etc.)

Risk of the transmission of diseases (toxoplasmosis, neosporosis, pseudo rage, contamination of the environment by salmonella, etc.)

Best for dog nutrition is a compromise between the two views. Meat-based dry food without unnecessary fillers can be found in most animal feed stores. With the occasional feeding of fresh meat, you will meet all of your pet's needs. All your Dog's food should always be sugar-free!

BARF for dogs - what is it?

"Biologically appropriate raw feeding."

A few years ago, BARF was still a nutritional method for exotic animals - meanwhile, "biologically appropriate raw feeding" has earned a permanent place in today's dog nutrition.

What is BARF?

BARF describes the raw feeding of dogs based on their original diet as carnivores, meat-eaters. From fresh meat, offal, vegetables, vitamin and mineral supplements, an attempt is made to imitate the wild dog's natural prey as much as possible.

## Why BARF?

Like any feeding method, raw feeding has many opponents and supporters. Dog friends who are convinced of the BARF report healthy teeth due to intensive chewing on fresh meat, shiny fur, improvement of chronic diseases such as osteoarthritis and growth problems, and a strong tendon and ligament system. Raw food is tailored to the individual Dog. It does not contain any fillers or preservatives - no wonder that this is an advantage, especially for sick dogs and those with special nutritional requirements!

## BARF - what should be considered?

If you want to feed your Dog with self-made raw meals, you are not only allowed to feed muscle meat - deficiency symptoms are guaranteed here! So that your Dog gets everything he needs, offal, vegetable components, vitamins, and minerals should be precisely calculated and weighed. For this reason, it is a complex and demanding feeding method. Fortunately, many dog food manufacturers and butchers are meeting the growing demand. So-called "Convenience BARF" products are put together directly by the manufacturer or butcher, frozen, and only need to be thawed and fed fresh by the dog owner. The zooplus dog magazine contains everything you need to pay attention to when it comes to baref puppies.

**Barfen for beginners**

Estimate effort and gather information:

Barfen is a complex feeding method. You must always plan to buy and store raw meat. Also, the feed must be precisely calculated. It is best to have the Dog checked out by the vet beforehand so that you know exactly which nutrients your Dog needs to consume. You should also find out about the various BARF methods to assess which variant suits your Dog best.

Pay attention to the choice of meat:

You should find out what meat you are feeding your Dog. For example, not all innards are suitable for barfing, because the liver and kidneys, in particular, contain harmful substances and should therefore be fed at most once a week. Pork can also be dangerous for the animals as it can transmit the Aujeszky virus, which is fatal for dogs.

Be careful when feeding bones!

Always take care not to split the bones you are feeding. This will avoid injuring your Dog.

A varied diet:

Muscle meat should not be the only component of the feed. Also offal, bones, oils, fruit, and vegetables (both pureed). Caution: some fruits and vegetables are poisonous.

# CHAPTER 2: CALCULATING THE AMOUNT OF FOOD FOR DOGS: IT'S THAT EASY

Proper nutrition for a dog also includes an amount of precisely tailored food to the four-legged friend.

Nowadays, it is not that easy to keep track of the different ways of feeding. If you opt for complete feed, you can easily read the recommended amount of feed from the packaging. But how do you calculate the amount of food in dogs if you want to bark or combine different feed materials? Fortunately, you can easily determine your four-legged friend's energy requirements with the help of a few formulas.

How much food does a dog need?

The answer to this question cannot be given a general answer, as your Dog's nutritional needs depend on various factors. If you want to calculate the exact amount of food for dogs, you must therefore take the following parameters into account:

- the age of your Dog
- the breed of Dog
- the weight in kilograms

Is it a very sporty dog , or is it a mother during pregnancy or suckling?

For a healthy dog diet, it is important that you also have a good balance of energy and proteins in the food ration in addition to the content of vitamins and minerals. You can read the ingredients of single and complete feed directly on the packaging.

In the case of complete feed, the weight-dependent amount of feed can also be found on the packaging. If you want to feed straight feed instead, you have to calculate the correct amount yourself. This is very easy with the help of the following formulas.

**Calculate the amount of food for adult dogs**

Adult dogs no longer grow, but they have a higher energy expenditure than older dogs. Fortunately, there are some formulas for calculating the correct amount of food for dogs individually.

What are the energy requirements of adult dogs?

The energy required is given in megajoules (MJ) or kilocalories (kcal). Using the Meyer and Zentek formula, you can calculate the average amount of energy your adult dog needs in a day:

Energy maintenance requirement of adult dogs = 0.52 MJ x kg 0.75 body weight.

Example: If your Dog weighs 20 kilograms, its energy requirement is calculated as follows: 0.52 MJ x 20 kg 0.75 = 4.91 MJ per day.

You can also use the following table as a guide:

| Body mass (kilograms) | Amount of energy (megajoules) | Amount of energy (kilocalories) |
|---|---|---|
| 5 | 1.74 | 415.87 |
| 10 | 2.92 | 697.90 |

| | | |
|---|---|---|
| 20 | 4.92 | 1175.91 |
| 30 | 6.67 | 1595.17 |
| 40 | 8.23 | 1967.02 |
| 50 | 9.78 | 2337.48 |

Protein requirements of adult dogs

Proteins are vital for dogs. They are present in all tissues and at the same time form the basis of important enzymes and hormones. You can calculate the average protein requirement for adult dogs using the following formula: The protein maintenance requirement of adult dogs corresponds to about 5g of crude protein x kg 0.75 body weight .

This results in the following protein table:

| Body weight (kilograms) | Amount of protein (grams) |
|---|---|
| 5 | 16 |

| | |
|---|---|
| 10 | 28 |
| $20^{th}$ | 47 |
| $30^{th}$ | 64 |
| 40 | 79 |
| 50 | 94 |

How is the amount of food calculated for sporty dogs?

If your dog is very athletic and has to cover long distances during the day, he will use more energy than a normal family dog. Therefore, in addition to the maintenance requirement, you must also calculate the power requirement.

The power requirement for the energy required for increased activity is calculated as follows: 0.56 MJ x kg 0.75 body weight.

For example, if your dog weighs 10 kilograms, it needs around 3.15 megajoules per day. That corresponds to about 752.87 kilocalories.

The need for proteins increases only slightly, however.

## How much food do pregnant bitches need?

If you have a bitch who is pregnant and is in the second half of her gestation period, she needs 1.5 times the energy maintenance requirement. A bitch weighing 20 kilograms needs about 7.38 megajoules per day.

The need for proteins is also increasing enormously. Therefore you have to add 0.5 times the protein maintenance requirement on average.

## How to calculate the amount of food for lactating bitches

The mother dog must produce a lot of milk while suckling. The exact amount depends on the number and size of the puppies to be looked after. On average, the energy requirement per puppy increases as follows:

| Number of puppies | P |
|---|---|
| 1 | 1.5 times the |

| | |
|---|---|
| $4^{th}$ | 2-fold main |
| $8^{th}$ | 3-fold main |

Example: Your bitch has given birth to eight puppies and weighs 20 kilograms. Therefore, your energy requirement is composed as follows: 4.92 MJ maintenance requirement x 3 = 14.76 MJ per day.

The protein requirement increases only slightly.

How much dog food does a puppy need?

Puppies grow quickly in the first few months. During this time, your organs need many nutrients, which they initially obtain from breast milk and the age of three months from solid food.

The formula for small breed puppies is 0.66 MJ x 0.75 kg body weight.

On the other hand, puppies of larger dog breeds require 0.75 MJ x kg 0.75 bodyweights.

Although young dogs need a relatively large amount of food, they must not be overfed. If the feed is too rich in carbohydrates, it can lead to obesity, growth disorders in the skeleton, and organ damage.

Puppies also need a lot of protein as they grow. However, this depends heavily on the particular breed of dog and must be considered individually. Proteins made from high-quality, essential amino acids are best. These have a higher value and are better implemented by the body than non-essential amino acids.

To provide puppies with everything they need for their growth, it is advisable to feed them suitable puppy food. You can also find more about puppy nutrition in the zooplus magazine.

## How do I calculate the amount of food for old dogs?

From around six years of age, dogs are considered seniors. From this point on, they need less energy to supply their life-sustaining organs. The factor 0.5 for adult dogs is reduced to 0.45 for senior dogs.

To calculate the correct amount of food for older dogs, the energy formula is now: 0.45 MJ x kg 0.75 bodyweight.

How many times a day should I feed my dogs?

Puppies' digestive systems still have to adapt to solid food in the first few months. Therefore, you should feed young four-legged friends more often than older dogs. It is usually enough to feed puppies three to four times a day. Make sure to reduce the rations at the same time.

When the dog is fully grown, it is sufficient to feed it only once or twice a day. You should make sure to offer the food at similar times of the day. Also, don't forget to include treats in your dog's amount of food.

**Ten Rules For Ideal Dog Nutrition**

Rule 1: Feed adult dogs once a day

From the age of about half a year, the requirements for dog nutrition change. Your darling is fully grown, and feeding once a day is completely sufficient. Use the meat-based dry food for this. There should always be something to drink with it. An additional, small snack such as a treat is allowed. If you want to offer snacks regularly, you should use meat-based, grain-free, soy-free, and gluten-free alternatives.

### Rule 2: adjust dog nutrition to age

Puppies younger than two months are given six servings per day. After that, the meals are slowly reduced to four. If the young animal does not manage to empty its bowl, you should remove the remains. Pay attention to regular feeding times! At three to four months, you can further reduce the rations to two times a day. Pay attention to how much your little darling is eating and adjust the bowl's amount of food accordingly.

### Rule 3: Feed regularly

Regular feeding is better for both owners and dogs. The organism can adapt to this and thus facilitate digestion. The routine in everyday life also ensures a balanced nature of the dogs, and the dreaded overfeeding is avoided.

Rule 4: Noon is the best time

Ideally, you will be fed at lunchtime when you also have your meal—a big advantage: your dog is distracted and does not beg at the table. Only give him what he normally gives up. If there is still anything left over, the remains will be removed as soon as your dog turns away from the bowl.

Rule 5: variety in taste

When feeding dogs, you should not switch between wet and dry food or the manufacturer. The different composition of the contents can lead to digestive problems with your four-legged friend. The flavor variety can be changed within the same manufacturer. Mixing different flavors is also possible without hesitation.

Rule 6: The dosage of dog food can only be done individually

The correct dosage of dog food is different for every dog. It depends on many factors: Age, size or weight, breed, and activity of your dog should be taken into account. Changes in the coat, the fat layer, or the digestion can also be important indicators. Also, based on how much your dog typically eats. Leftovers are removed, and your darling seems to be still hungry, can also be portioned.

## Rule 7: Feed hygienically and at the right temperature

Raw meat and wet food, in particular, must not be too cold or warm; your dog can tolerate them best at room temperature. Another problem with these forms of feeding is hygiene. When preparing it at home, germs or bacteria can quickly develop. On the other hand, meat-based dry food is always at the right temperature, and neither bacteria nor germs can settle without moisture.

## Rule 8: The right drink

You should only give your fresh dog water to drink. Neither carbonic acid nor other beverages intended for humans may be administered. It is best to always have fresh water available to your darling. Dry food only contains 10% moisture, so more should be drunk.

### Rule 9: Give your dog some rest while digesting

After eating, your dog needs rest for digestion. Walks and other activities should therefore be postponed! Then the individual vitamins, nutrients, and minerals are better absorbed by the organism. Also, the break promotes a balanced nature in your dog.

### Rule 10: Fasting regularly

Your dog shouldn't get anything to eat on the weekly fasting day. That won't bother him any further, as a hunting wolf is not always successful. Fasting is, therefore, your dog's nature. Unnecessary reserves are thus reduced. Even if the animal does not eat a meal on its initiative, there is still no need to worry. However, if food intake continues to be denied or is abnormally low, you should see your vet.

**The optimal dog nutrition**

For a species-appropriate, healthy, and varied dog nutrition, all of the above rules must be followed. Especially for four-legged friends who live in the apartment, dry food is the most hygienic and simplest solution. The animal's health is also taken into account with meat-based products without grain or other vegetable additives. If you observe your dog's eating behavior closely, you will quickly discover their preferences for different flavors. In all attempts to convince yourself of other dog nutrition methods, you should keep in mind: Your dog is 98.8% a wolf and only 0.2% a pet.

# CHAPTER 3: BARF OR CONVENTIONAL DOG FOOD?

Which feeding method is best for your dog?

Dry, wet, or do you prefer fresh and raw? Our four-legged friends' opinions about the right feeding method are as diverse as the selection of types of food in stores. But is Barfen healthier? Does wet food taste better, and is dry food cheaper? We will show you the main advantages and disadvantages of the various feeding methods.

The feeding method that is equally best for all dogs does not exist to come to the point. Whether BARF, dry or wet food - every dog food has its advantages and disadvantages. In principle, you can feed your dog healthily with all three variants and ensure an optimal supply of energy and nutrients.

A question of taste?

The question of the best feeding method is less a question of right or wrong than a question of your possibilities and demands. Which food does my dog tolerate best? How much time do I have to prepare the dog food? Does my dog have illnesses that require a special diet? And can I even afford the chosen form of feeding? To make this personal decision a little easier for you, we would first like to explain the differences between dry, wet, and raw feeding and which points speak for and against the three different administration types.

## The three categories of dog food

Whether it is a supermarket, pet shop, or the Internet - no other pet has such a huge range of food as it is for dogs. Whether a puppy, adult or senior dog, whether sporty or overweight dog, whether allergy sufferer or sick dog, whether large or small breed - there is a special food for each of our four-legged friends. No wonder that especially beginners are often overwhelmed with this offer. It helps to first consider a few facts about the different types of food. A distinction is usually made between three different categories of dog food:

- Dried animal food
- Wet or moist food
- BARF (fresh raw feed)

Interesting facts about dry food, wet food, and BARFs

With classic dry food, dried and ground raw materials are broken down by heat and pressed into so-called croquettes, usually available in large kilo bags and have a low to medium shelf life. On the other hand, the raw materials are filled directly into hermetically sealed cans and heated after being crushed and mixed in the case of moist or wet feed. As a result, wet food has a softer consistency and a more intense taste, and a comparatively high water and protein content. By heating in the closed can, the contents are preserved for a very long time.

As the third form of dog nutrition, the so-called barfen has established itself in the last few years, in which unprocessed (raw) fresh meat is put in the food bowl with raw, mostly pureed fruit and vegetables. The abbreviation BARF originally stood for "Born-again raw feeders" and later changed to "Bone and Raw Food". In German, the term is now usually translated as "biologically appropriate raw feeding." Made in the 1990s by the Australian vetIan Bilinghurst, who played a key role in developing the BARF method, is based on the natural diet of wolves. With the rations of raw fresh meat, offal, bones, vegetables, fruit, and nuts, it roughly imitates the wolf's prey, which consists of bones and meat and their stomach contents with processed berries and plants.

**Advantages of dry food**

Each of these three feeding methods has its advantages and disadvantages, and so every dog owner has to weigh himself up, which criteria are most important to him personally.

Storage and practical handling are undoubtedly one of the greatest advantages of dry food. The light kilo bags can be bought in advance and easily allocated. Anyone who is often out and about with their dog will appreciate the simple and clean portioning. The type of packaging also keeps the amount of waste very limited. Dry food is certainly the fastest and easiest solution for trips and trips.

Another advantage can be that dry food has a very high nutrient content, even in small quantities. Compared to wet food, the portions are significantly smaller. Besides, the nutrients are in production due to the heat process already open-minded and ensures very high digestibility. Depending on the size and density, the dry kibble stimulates the dogs to chew. The kibble size can be selected depending on the size of the dog and its teeth.

**Disadvantages of dry food**

At the same time, however, the croquettes' shape does not allow any conclusions to be drawn about the raw materials used. The associated uncertainty about the quality of the ingredients is certainly the greatest disadvantage of dry food. It is advisable to read the declaration on the packaging carefully because many varieties have an extremely high proportion of carbohydrates, which can quickly lead to obesity in dogs. Insufficient fluid intake can also be problematic. Since dry food has a very low moisture content, owners must make sure that their dogs also drink enough water.

## Benefits of wet food

Wet food consists of around 70 to 80 percent liquid. Wet food is therefore particularly suitable for dogs who drink very little. And even picky eaters like wet food have a more intense taste, often better than dry food. Small breeds, in particular, prefer the soft consistency of the food. Also, the proportion of animal proteins essential for the animals is usually higher in moist feed than in dry feed, for example. Heating in closed packaging such as cans or pouches also ensures a very long shelf life. Also, as with dry food, the ingredients are broken down by the heating, which positively affects digestibility.

## Disadvantages of wet food

Similar to dry food, you should pay close attention to the declaration of wet food so that you can see which ingredients have been used. About the quality of the animal proteins, there can be big differences between the manufacturers, but this is also the case with dry food and ready-to-use barf meals. The proportion of meat and animal by-products should be balanced. Dog owners often cite the short shelf life of opened containers for wet food as a disadvantage - once open, the food spoils quickly. Others also find the stronger smell of wet food unpleasant. Another disadvantage is the large amount of packaging waste, which is mainly caused by cans.

**Benefits of the BARF method**

In contrast to classic dry or wet food, barfe is considered more natural, more appropriate to the species, and healthier, especially by fans of this feeding method. Whether the BARF method is healthier has not yet been scientifically proven. Still, since the rations are put together themselves, owners can cater more to their dog's individual needs. For example, food components that trigger allergies can simply be replaced by another food component in allergy sufferers. Changes such as the dog's size, weight, or level of activity can also be taken into account in a more individualized manner. Besides, the use of individual food components, i.e., fresh meat and fresh fruit and vegetables, enables a better assessment of the quality.

**Disadvantages of the BARF method**

One of the problems with barfing lies in the way you put your products together. To adapt the rations as optimally as possible to the dog's individual nutritional needs, a lot of knowledge and experience is required. An incorrect distribution of nutrients can lead to overweight or underweight and severe deficiency symptoms or oversupply, which leads to serious health risks. Pathogens contained in raw meat, fish, and eggs are another risk. Raw pork should not be fed to dogs and cats. Most bacteria are killed during cooking, but they can survive in the freezer for a very long time and even multiply during the thawing process.

Summary: All advantages and disadvantages at a glance

| BENEFITS |
| --- |

| | |
|---|---|
| Dried animal food | cheap price<br>medium durability<br>easy to use and easy to take with you when traveling<br>high nutrient requirement<br>allows smaller portions (à better digestibility)<br>easy storage<br>little packaging waste |
| Wet food | high liquid content (improvemen of the water balance of "little drinkers")<br>more intense taste<br>soft consistency is often preferred by small dogs<br>mostly high proportion of animal proteins<br>very long shelf life |
| Barf | The use of fresh products allows a good assessment of the quality<br>Rations can be tailored individual to the dog's needs<br>No undesirable substances in the feed |

Looking at the table, you can see that the three different feeding methods' advantages and disadvantages are fairly evenly distributed. The question of which dosage form is the best or healthiest for the dog can, therefore, hardly be answered across the board. After all, dogs - just like us humans - are individuals and have different needs, tastes, and demands. The decision of which food is right for your dog can only be made personally. Do not be unsettled by other dog owners' opinions, in Internet forums, or on the dog park. The important thing is that you and your dog are happy with your choice.

It is not the form, the content that matters.

First and foremost, the selected food must, of course, meet your dog's nutritional needs and provide him with everything he needs for healthy development. Whether this is the case depends less on the form of the feed than on its content. If you take a closer look at the individual ingredients and their quality, you can feed your dog sufficiently and healthily with both classic dog food and the BARF method. Your dog's age, weight, size, and activity level must be taken into account when choosing a food. Illnesses and possible allergies also play a decisive role. And of course, personal circumstances will also influence your decision. Think carefully about how much time you can spend on food preparation,

Look for the best solution for you and your dog.

Also, talk to your veterinarian about the different feeding options. Perhaps a mix of dry and wet food or BARF and conventional food is also a good idea. For beginners who would like to barf, the portion-wise packaged BARF menus offered on the Internet can also be a practical solution. One thing is certain: as long as the energy and nutrient supply is guaranteed and your dog is healthy and vital, there is no wrong method.

# CHAPTER 4: DIFFERENT DOGS AND THEIR DIETS

## Bernese Mountain Dog nutrition

What should I put attention on?

Robust, vigilant, talented in pulling a wagon and driving animals, and a versatile farm dog - that was the breeding goal for the Bernese Mountain Dog at the beginning of the twentieth century. He comes from Bern's area in Switzerland, where his nickname "Dürrbächler" originates from an inn near Riggisberg in the canton of Bern. It is believed that St. Bernard, Newfoundland, and German Shepherd types were crossed.

The Bernese Mountain Dog weighs around 39 to 50 kilos (males) or 36 to 45 kilos (females) with a shoulder height of up to 70 centimeters. This means that the dogs belong to the physically strong, well-built breeds they like to show in their everyday tasks. They reach the age of 8 to 10 years; in some cases, the animals get significantly older.

The Bernese Mountain Dog's fur is long, soft, and smooth and black with brownish-red and white markings. Because of their thick coat, they are troubled by hot weather. In cooler temperatures, however, they feel very comfortable.

In addition to being used as a self-confident farm dog, the Bernese Mountain Dog complements every family in an enriching way due to its friendly, good-natured, and people-related nature. His pronounced alertness without aggression and his ability to get along well with children round off this character. Only males can react indignantly to their peers, especially in their territory. When dealing with people, the dog reacts calmly by observing calmly and only intervening when necessary. Its stimulus threshold is accordingly extremely high. The Bernese Mountain Dog hardly has any hunting instinct, so that it does not tend to stray, and after a good basic educationFreewheel is possible without any problems. This is important as it requires a lot of exercise and activity. He also has to see the point in the commands and tasks given to him. In other words: a Bernese Mountain Dog can sometimes seem stubborn.

The dog breed is not very suitable for activities that require agility and speed. However, it can be used excellently for dog work, rescue, or tracking training and areas where anticipatory obedience is required. The animals also feel very comfortable in the therapy area and as school dogs.

## Right from the start - healthy nutrition for a Bernese Mountain Dog puppy

The Bernese Mountain Dog is one of the tall dogs. For puppies of this breed, it is important to ensure that the food's amount is appropriate for healthy growth. Because of the excessive supply of energy in the food, the dog's genetically determined final weight can be reached earlier than intended or even higher. The skeleton is not yet sufficiently stable for this, which can lead to malpositions of the limbs. To get a strong and stable skeleton, adequate energy intake and a balanced supply of minerals, especially calcium and phosphorus, are essential for Bernese Mountain Dog puppies.

For a Bernese Mountain Dog puppy's healthy growth, you should pay attention to a needs-based and balanced proportion of energy, minerals, trace elements, and vitamins.

Feeding recommendations for puppy food is based on the puppy's current weight and the expected weight as an adult dog. You can use the weight of the same-sex parent animal as a guide. The amount of food also depends on the puppy's level of activity. A cozy puppy doesn't need the same amount of food as a very active puppy.

**Big and strong - healthy nutrition for Bernese Mountain Dogs**

The Bernese Mountain Dog is valued as a family dog because of its good-natured temperament. He is also kind and affectionate toward children. Since they are also very adaptive and vigilant, they are also used as companion dogs. The Bernese Mountain Dog does not shy away from physical work, making it an ideal draft dog and tracker, which also proves itself a rescue and disaster dog. Depending on the Bernese Mountain Dog's lifestyle, its needs and the demands on its food differ. When used as a draft dog or tracker, the need for energy and food is high. However, the Bernese Mountain Dog also enjoys being active as a family dog by playing and romping with the children or through sports programs and extensive hikes. Every single dog has certain characteristics and, thus, individual nutritional requirements. The nutrient and energy requirements of a dog differ depending on their size, weight, and activity. Also, the Bernese Mountain Dog's common diseases, such as obesity and joint problems, should be taken into account in the diet.

The diet of a Bernese Mountain Dog should be switched to adult dog food after it is fully grown. The more sporty and active the dog, the more carbohydrates the food can contain for energy supply. However, with cozy and calm dogs, you should pay attention to a moderate amount of carbohydrates so that they do not become overweight. The fat content should also be in the medium range. In addition to the level of activity and composition of the feed, the feed amount is also decisive for the weight. The giving of treats and rewards should not be ignored. The number of treats should be deducted from the daily ration. Whether you choose a suitable wet or dry food or combine both types of food,

## The best of years - healthy aging with the right diet

Like humans, dogs also age. We all know older dog owners with a gray beard. But it's not just the coat that changes in older dogs. The rest of the body also shows signs of old age. Associated with these physical changes are other nutritional requirements for the dog. As the activity of senior dogs decreases, their energy requirements decrease at the same time. The energy supply in the feed should, therefore, be reduced if necessary so that the senior does not gain weight. Some older dogs may also have a poor sense of smell and taste, which is why a particularly tasty food can be beneficial. Special food for older dogs addresses the nutritional needs of old age.

## St. Bernard diet

St. Bernard dogs are among the most popular family dogs. With a height at the withers of 65 to 90 cm and a weight of 55 to 80 kilograms, they are also among the largest and heaviest breeds of dogs.

In the past, they were mainly used as working and rescue dogs.

What should I put attention on?

The massive Saint Bernard got its name from the first records that reveal that the dogs were used for protection in a hospice that monks founded on the great St. Bernhard pass in Switzerland in the 11th century as a place of refuge for travelers and pilgrims. Since then, the St. Bernard has been used as a companion, rescue, and avalanche dog in snow and fog to rescue lost travelers. Today, however, due to their heavy physique, the Saint Bernard dogs are only suitable to a limited extent as rescue dogs, but they are popular for care, rehabilitation, or companion dogs. Together with the Bernese Mountain Dog, they are among the most famous Swiss dog breeds.

There are two varieties in the appearance of the St. Bernard. One with short, dense, smooth, and close-fitting fur, the other has medium-length outer hair. In both cases, the fur is red and white with white paws, chest, and tail tip. A compact and muscular body, an imposing head, and an attentive facial expression round off the overall sublime appearance.

As a rescue dog, Saint Bernard stood out primarily because of his good-natured, watchful, balanced and reliable nature. Hardly anything can upset him so that he is even open to strangers and usually likes to be petted and touched by strangers and children. Hardly any other dog is so tolerant, balanced, and fond of children. For this reason, Saint Bernard, although he is an impressive figure due to his size, is ideal as a family dog, especially since he uncompromisingly and extremely effectively defends his family and his kingdom without ever losing control (provided he is well behaved). He is also very affectionate and needs a lot of contact with people and other dogs.

**Giant dog - still very small**

The St. Bernard can be counted among the large dogs or Molossians. Especially with large and heavy dog breeds, it is particularly important to ensure that the energy content (calories) in the food is needs-based for the respective puppy. If the energy content is too high, there is a risk that they will grow too quickly. As a result, the genetically determined final weight for each dog can be reached too early, so that the skeleton is not yet aligned for this weight. Serious malpositions of the limbs can be the result. To prevent this mistake, St. Bernard puppies should be given a feed that provides them with minerals (especially calcium and phosphorus), trace elements, vitamins, and energy as required. Nothing stands in the way of the gentle giant's healthy growth.

When it comes to feeding recommendations, the puppy's current weight and the expected weight as an adult dog should be taken into account. To estimate the expected weight, you use the weight of the same-sex parent animal. When dividing the amount of food, the puppy's age and activity are also taken into account.

**The gentle giant - nutrition of the adult St. Bernard**

Due to its size and mass alone, the St. Bernard is not one of the breeds characterized by a strong need for exercise. Nowadays, Saint Bernard rarely fulfills its original activity as a rescue dog due to its physique, which has changed considerably compared to then. As a result, St. Bernard's nutritional needs have changed considerably. Today, the St. Bernard is considered a balanced companion dog that is not upset so quickly. His diet should be adapted to his body mass and activity. Problems with the joints affect the body even more because of size and weight. Unfortunately, the St. Bernard is now more prone to hip dysplasia. A diet with moderate energy content and high-quality ingredients can prevent obesity and joint problems: the energy requirements and the amount of food for a dog decrease determine the height, weight, and activity.

Especially with such a large breed as the St. Bernard, which reaches a high final weight in adulthood, an optimal diet with a balanced and needs-based composition is necessary. After the St. Bernard is fully grown, the diet should be switched to a diet for adult dogs. The giving of treats and snacks should not be disregarded in the daily feeding. The number of treats fed should be deducted from the daily ration of food.

## Aging healthily with proper nutrition

As with humans, older dogs show the signs of the times. Since St. Bernard dogs, as giant breeds, have a shorter life expectancy than smaller dog breeds, they start aging earlier. The dog's metabolism changes and with it the nutritional needs. The energy requirement decreases as the activity decreases. You should choose a food with suitable energy content; reduced fat content is also recommended to control weight and increased fiber content for digestion. The sense of smell and taste can decrease, which is why tasty food is recommended. To support the St. Bernard Seniors' immune system, senior foods usually contain a high proportion of antioxidants.

## Chihuahua diet

The Chihuahua is lively, vigilant, restless, and very brave according to the breed standard and is considered the smallest breed globally. The Chihuahua needs a lot of attention and is picky about how to give it affection. The Chihuahua diet should not be ignored either. We explain what needs to be considered.

How can I feed my Chihuahua?

In addition to care and care, a needs-based diet is a particularly important support for a good start in healthy dog life. You should pay attention to a needs-based and balanced proportion of energy, minerals, trace elements, and vitamins in puppy food. In contrast to large breeds, there is a greater risk of oversupply with small breeds.

Feeding puppy food recommendations are based on the puppy's current weight and the expected weight as an adult dog. The weight of same-sex parents can be used as a guide. Also, the amount of food depends on the puppy's level of activity.

Chihuahua diet: what food can I give my puppy?

For a puppy of the breed Chihuahua, the puppy food Royal Canin Chihuahua Puppy is recommended as dry food and as wet food Royal Canin Mini Puppy. The feeding amount for puppies should always be divided into several meals per day. Also, the dog must always have fresh water available.

## Small dog, big: feeding the adult Chihuahua

For adult Chihuahuas, the diet should be switched to food for adult dogs. Although Chihuahuas are not known to become overweight, one should still keep an eye on their favorite weight.

The Chihuahua is one of the toy breeds with a short snout. Warmer temperatures are unfavorable for him and should therefore be better avoided. High body weight could exacerbate this problem.

Whether you offer your Chihuahua wet or dry food or mix both types of food is up to you. Most of the time, the dog decides for himself by his preferences.

When it comes to dry food, we recommend small croquettes adapted to the teeth of small dogs. Besides, dry food is easy to store and generates less packaging waste than wet food.

These dry food croquettes are also well suited as a reward or for training. Alternatively, you can also use various small snacks for this. However, you must subtract the number of treats from the daily ration of the feed. Otherwise, it can easily lead to obesity.

Wet food is often very popular because it is tastier than dry food. The fluid intake is also higher with wet food, as the moisture content is usually over 70 percent.

**Diet for Chihuahua Seniors**

An older and small dog needs a diet that is tailored to its age and size, as the aging process brings about physical changes—metabolism and activity decrease. An appropriately adapted diet with high acceptance and palatability can support the well-being of an older Chihuahua.

He stays in shape for as long as possible, his food should be adapted to the specific signs of age and thus optimally promote healthy aging.

**German shepherd diet**

If you think of German dog breeds, you probably immediately think of it: the German Shepherd. This is certainly not only due to its size and conspicuous presence but also because we encounter us again and again as a service and companion dog in everyday life. At the end of the 19th century, the German Shepherd Dog Association was founded, which has since established the dog breed's breeding guidelines. The German Shepherd Dog was bred out of the Central German and South German lofts of the herding dogs at that time: The aim was to create a working dog with high performance.

With a height at the withers of 55 to 65 centimeters (bitches up to 60 centimeters), the sporty herding dogs weigh about 22 to 40 kilograms (bitches up to 32 kilograms). The physique is muscular but slim and elongated. At around 13 years of age, they reach an impressive age for large dogs. The robust and short coat in black with yellow to red-brown signs and a thick undercoat requires little maintenance.

Agile shepherds love sports such as running, cycling, or agility, as well as long walks in all weathers. As herding dogs, German Shepherds have a strong sense of family and protective instinct, although they are generally fond of children. The animals are strong-nerved, self-confident and courageous, fearless, and ready to fight in threatening situations.

The innate obedience and the will to please his caregiver make German Shepherd's ideal candidates for dog sports and training become rescue, detection, or police dogs. Dogs of this breed are also ideal as guide dogs or companions for people with disabilities. When upbringing, the animals need a harsh tone, they like to learn through positive confirmation and cleverly placed rewards with simultaneous consistency. Thus trained, they are safe and loyal family members or partners in their hobby and work.

Unfortunately, joint diseases, especially of the hip ( hip dysplasia, HD ) and elbow, are relatively widespread in German shepherds. Affected animals are more or less restricted in their freedom of movement and suffer from pain. An HD control in the breed association and breeding value estimation methods are intended to contain the spread of hip dysplasia.

**German shepherd puppy diet**

The active German Shepherd is one of the large dogs. Puppies and young dogs of large breeds need food with moderate energy content adapted to their individual needs to not grow too quickly. It is particularly advisable to have a growth curve made for dogs of large breeds so that you can keep a close eye on healthy growth. The end weight of a dog, which is genetically determined, can be reached earlier than intended due to an excess of energy in the food and can even be higher. However, the musculoskeletal system is not yet sufficiently stable. This overload can cause misalignments of the limbs. As German Shepherds often struggle with joint diseases, appropriate feeding is particularly important for this breed.

The recommendations for the amount of food for a puppy are based on the one hand on the puppy's current weight and, on the other hand, on the expected weight as an adult dog. The expected weight is determined based on the weight of the same-sex parent animal. For a male, for example, the father's weight is used as a guide. Also, the level of activity must be taken into account in the amount of feed.

## Good food for your best friend: nutrition for adult German Shepherds

Whether the German Shepherd Dog is used as a rescue, detection, or police dog or lives as a loyal friend and companion in a family can impact its nutritional needs. Depending on the German Shepherd area and activity, the demands on its food differ. As a companion, rescue, tracker, or police dog, the need for energy in the food and food is rather high. As a family member, the German Shepherd Dog needs just as much activity for "mind and body," be it through sporting activities and extensive hikes or various types of games. Here, however, the need for energy in the feed is usually a little less than "on duty." But it is not just activity, race, and weight that create certain nutritional needs. Every dog has different characteristics and individual requirements.

After the German Shepherd has reached its adult weight and age, the diet should be switched to adult dogs' food. The level of activity should also be taken into account when choosing the food for adult dogs. For inactive and sporty dogs, the food may contain more carbohydrates as an energy source. In contrast, less active dogs should have a moderate amount of carbohydrates to not become overweight. Especially with a breed like the German Shepherd, which often suffers from diseases of the joints, obesity must be avoided at all costs to not aggravate this problem. In addition to the dog's level of activity and the composition of the food, the amount of food is, of course, also decisive for the weight. Treats and rewards should be taken into account and deducted from the daily ration of the feed. Whether you look at choosing a suitable oneWet food or dry food or a combination of both is a matter of taste for the dog and the owner.

**The best friend in the prime: food for seniors**

As the dogs get older, their bodies and metabolism change, making the demands on their diet: the energy requirement usually drops because the dogs are no longer as active as before. So you should reduce the energy supply depending on the level of activity in the feed so that the senior does not gain weight. Besides, some older dogs have a poor sense of smell and taste, so a particularly tasty food can be advantageous.

**The French Bulldog Diet**

The short-nosed French Bulldog is dependent on a special diet due to its anatomy and physiology. Due to the shortened nose and thus also very rudimentary turbinates, the temperature regulation and the air supply of the French Bulldog are impaired. This is a significant handicap, especially at higher temperatures. Besides, the Bully is anything but a marathon runner due to its physique. To not aggravate its impairments, appropriate body weight is very important for the well-being of the French Bulldog.

The breed probably originally descended from the English Bulldog and was used, among other things, for dog fights. English lacemakers emigrated to France at the end of the 19th century when large lace factories were established. They took these bulldogs to France and bred the French Bulldog here by crossing other breeds. In Germany, the friendly, happy, and bright dog has been an absolute fashion breed for several years.

**Healthy nutrition - an important prerequisite for a healthy dog life**

The French Bulldog is one of the small breeds of dogs and can reach a weight of approx. 8-14 kg, depending on their height. With Bully puppies, you should pay attention to an appropriate amount of energy in the food; otherwise, they can reach a higher weight than intended and unstable bones can develop. This can lead to misalignment of the limbs if the physique is already compact.

For a good start to a healthy dog's life, you should ensure that your puppy food contains a balanced proportion of energy, minerals, trace elements, and vitamins appropriate to your needs.

Feeding puppy food recommendations are based on the puppy's current weight and the expected weight as an adult dog. The weight of same-sex parents can be used as a guide. Also, the amount of food depends on the puppy's level of activity.

**In the prime of life - feeding a full-grown French Bulldog.**

For an adult Bully, the diet should be changed to food for adult dogs. The French Bulldog is prone to obesity. She loves walks over hill and dale but is not suitable for covering longer distances. It is better to let them romp around in the meadow than to go on long hikes. This is due to their anatomy, the stocky build, and the short snout with frequent breathing and temperature regulation problems.

Nevertheless, regular exercise is important to keep the animal fit and to prevent obesity. Croquettes from dry food or low-fat snacks are suitable as treats because they can always be rewarded. The amount of treats is best subtracted from the daily ration of the feed. The fat and carbohydrate content in the feed should be moderate to keep the Bully's weight in check. Wet food is particularly suitable, as the amount of moisture to be fed higher than with dry food, and the hungry dog's stomach is more full. Besides, wet food's energy content is lower than that of dry food, which can be particularly beneficial for dogs that tend to be overweight. Liquid absorption is higher with wet food, as the moisture content is usually over 70%.

Liquid absorption is higher with wet food, as the moisture content is usually over 70%. Liquid absorption is higher with wet food, as the moisture content is usually over 70%.

## Nutrition for elderly bullies

As in humans, physical changes occur with age in our animal friends. Thus the requirements for nutrition change. The energy requirement decreases due to the reduced exercise of senior dogs. Likewise, the sense of smell and taste decreases. It is therefore advisable to give a particularly tasty and energy-reduced feed to support the elderly Bullys.

The diet of the Australian Shepherd

What should I put attention on?

Although its name suggests otherwise, the lively Australian Shepherd does not come from the continent Down Under, but from the USA. The forerunner of the breed was a herding dog from the Basque Country. In the steadily growing demand for Australian wool in the 19th century, this was imported from Australia by American sheep farmers to accompany immigrating Basque shepherds and their herds. Back then, the Basques were professional shepherds who moved with their animals from continent to continent. So they got around in many countries, resulting in the long-haired collie, short-haired collie, German Shepherd, Pyrenees shepherd, Australian cattle dog, and Australian kelpiewere involved in the development of the "Aussie," as it is also known. The breed reached Europe in the 1970s, and it was not recognized by the FCI (Fédération Cynologique Internationale) until 1996.

The Australian Shepherd is still today characterized by its lively and intelligent character with a high level of guarding instinct, especially as herding, working, or companion dog, and is often trained and used accordingly, such as therapy, guide, or rescue dog. Due to his friendly and balanced nature, he is also particularly suitable for a family dog and children.

When purchasing an Australian Shepherd, it should be noted that, on the one hand, he is usually fixated on people and does not like to be left alone for long. On the other hand, he needs regular activities and tasks and demands them; dogs of this breed love long walks, agility, or exercises in the dog park.

Outwardly, the breed is very attractive with up to sixteen permitted, individual color variations for medium-length, coarse hair. The basic colors, however, are black and red. In its maximum 13 to 15 years of life, the "Aussie" has a height at the withers of 51 to 58 cm (males) or 46 to 53 cm (females) and is therefore of medium size. Clear features of the Australian Shepherd are, on the one hand, the frequently occurring two-tone eyes, the slightly rounded tips of the ears, and a friendly face.

### Healthy growth for active dogs

The Australian Shepherd can be described as a medium-sized breed of dog. Puppies of this breed should be fed a moderate amount in energy content to prevent them from growing too quickly. Excessive energy supply in the food in puppies can mean that the genetically determined final weight is reached earlier than intended or is higher.

However, the skeleton is not yet sufficiently stable. This can result in misalignment of the limbs. Aussie puppies, therefore, need an energy intake that is adapted to the respective activity level as well as a balanced supply of minerals, especially calcium and phosphorus, trace elements, and vitamins.

Feeding puppy food recommendations are based on the puppy's current weight and the expected weight as an adult dog. The weight of the same-sex parent animal serves as a guideline. Besides, the amount of food is divided according to the puppy's level of activity.

Use on four paws - even better with the right diet.

The Australian Shepherd is a lively and bright dog. Since it needs a lot of activity, it is suitable as a herding and companion dog, and it is also used as a therapy, guide, or rescue dog. The demands on the food differ depending on the area of

application of the dog. But it is not just used and breeds that bring certain requirements with them. Every single dog has its own needs and thus individual requirements for nutrition. A dog's nutritional needs vary based on size, weight, and activity. When it comes to nutrition, you should also consider the more common diseases of the Australian Shepherd, such as allergies, obesity, and joint problems.

After the Aussie is fully grown, the diet should be changed to an adult dog diet. For active dogs, the food may contain more carbohydrates for energy production. In contrast, calm dogs should have a moderate carbohydrate content so that they do not become overweight. The fat content should also be in the medium range. In addition to the level of activity and composition of the feed, the amount fed is also decisive for weight. The giving of treats and rewards should be taken into account. The number of treats should be deducted from the daily ration. Whether you choose a suitable wet or dry food when choosing a food decides or combines both types of food is a matter of taste for the dog and the owner.

## Better to be healthy than rusty - nutrition for older dogs

Dogs are also getting on in years. Older dogs have different needs than young dogs. The physical changes make other demands on the diet. Physical changes associated with age have different nutritional requirements for senior dogs. As elderly dogs become less active, their energy needs to decrease. So you should reduce the energy supply in the feed so that the senior does not gain weight. Since some older dogs have a reduced sense of smell and taste, particularly tasty food can be advantageous.

**The diet of the Beagle**

For him, it is quantity rather than quality that counts.

When you talk about the Beagle, the first thing that comes to mind is its voracity. The Beagle's feeding behavior is famous, its cheerfulness, amiability, and social behavior are also discussed. Snoopy is probably the most famous representative of the Beagle breed. As a pack dog, the Beagle is easy on other dogs and extremely child-friendly.

He is gentle, attentive, adaptable, and always in a good mood, making him a popular family dog. Since he has always been a hunting dog, he will pursue his passion whenever he gets the opportunity. In addition to his intelligence, he also shows a considerable degree of stubbornness and perseverance. The Beagle, therefore, requires intensive and consistent training.

Originally the Beagle probably came from England or France and was bred from the larger Southern or Fox Shound. The origin of the name "Beagle" is also not established. It probably comes from the Old

English word "begle," Celtic "beag," or Old French "beigh." All three terms correspond to the word "small" and were used for all small pack dogs.

The Beagle is a hunting dog bred to be a hunted pack dog especially for hunting hares and rabbits on foot. Searching for wilderness trails and rummaging are still in his blood today. In selecting the hunting dogs, emphasis was placed on the fact that beagles eat everything and large quantities without problems and show as little aggression as possible. This origin as a pack dog explains the tendency to want to eat excessively.

**Right from the start - the beagle puppy's healthy diet**

The Beagle is one of the medium-sized dog breeds and, when fully grown, reaches a height of approx. 33 to 40 cm and, depending on size and gender, a weight of approx. 9-18 kg.

Since beagles are known to have a particularly large appetite, you should pay attention to an appropriate amount of energy in the food from a puppy's age. Together with the little Beagle's upbringing, you can train feeding habits so that you can counteract obesity now. However, some opinions say you should feed a beagle irregularly, otherwise it will cling to your heels whining at least an hour before the feeding event. Everyone must find the best method for themselves and their Beagle. Despite educational measures, one should never leave food unattended within reach of a beagle.

When feeding the beagle puppy, you should pay attention to a needs-based and balanced proportion of energy, minerals, trace elements, and vitamins in the food. You should feed a puppy three to four times a day; you can switch to feeding twice from about the time you change teeth.

The feeding recommendations for puppy food are based on the puppy's current weight and the expected adult weight. The weight of same-sex parents can be used as a guide. Besides, the amount of food depends on the puppy's level of activity.

What can I do for you? Feeding the adult beagle

When the Beagle is fully grown or after the change of teeth, the diet should be switched to adult dogs' food. The Beagle has higher demands on the quantity than the quality of its "daily bread." Uncomfortable specimens of this breed are a rare exception. The Beagle's eating behavior has its origins in its origin as a hunting and packs dog.

As a result of their hunting activity, beagles lost a lot of calories that they had to take in again in a short time. Therefore, it is the responsibility of the dog owner to ensure that the Beagle cuts a good figure. Since the Beagle is a very friendly dog and doesn't like to be alone, you can take him everywhere with you. He needs a lot of exercise and activity. This can be in the form of search games, tricks, mantrailing, and much more. Due to the intelligence and determination of the Beagle, there are hardly any limits.

Part of the daily food ration can be fed as a reward during training. This part may then no longer end up in the food bowl as a ration. Croquettes from dry food or low-fat snacks are suitable as treats.

Which food you give your darling depends on the one hand on the dog's preference. On the other hand, it should also suit the dog owner. All types of feed have their advantages. It is also possible to combine several types of food, such as wet food at home, dry food while training. The moisture content of wet food is higher than that of dry food, so the dog's stomach is more full and, therefore, more saturated. The energy content in wet food is usually lower than in dry food. Also, the fluid intake through wet food is higher than with dry food.

**Diet for Beagle Oldies**

An older dog has different needs than a young dog. The body is also changing, and with it, the demands on the senior dog's nutrition. Reduced movement and metabolism reduce the energy requirement. So you should lower the energy supply in the feed so that the senior does not gain weight. Since the sense of smell and taste also diminishes in older dogs, particularly tasty food can be an advantage, even for beagles.

## The Border Collie's diet

What should I put attention on?

Dog lovers immediately love the fascinating Border Collie with its friendly and equally clever nature. He is unique in his thirst for learning, enthusiasm for work, and always easy to lead. While the dogs in the house are considered lovable, calm, and affectionate, they convince in their original use, the herding of sheep, through their intelligence, the is shown through vigilance and attention. The athletic constitution rounds off the qualities as a herding and leisure dog.

With his keen sense, quick perception, and quick reactions, he can drive sheep in any direction, lead them through gates or isolate individual animals from the herd. As good as he is for herding work, he is still not a reliable watchdog, as he usually reacts neutrally and positively to strangers.

The graceful, well-proportioned dog breed originated in Great Britain. The hardworking dogs are descended from the previously bred medieval British herding dogs (collies) and later became a new breed in the so-called Border Counties, the border areas between Scotland and England. Because of this, they were given the breed name Border Collie in 1910.

The thick, mostly black and white outer hair of the Border Collies can appear in two variants: On the one hand, medium-length and wavy, on the other hand, stick-haired or short-haired, i.e., straight. Also, there is a soft, dense, and, therefore, weatherproof undercoat. The long hair creates a mane, trousers, and a flag, but the fur on the face, ears, front and rear legs is short and smooth. All colors are allowed, but white must never predominate. The Border Collie reaches a size of 45 to 55 cm and weighs between 13 and 22 kg.

Pure physical activity is not enough in the long run for the Border Collie, who moves elegantly and effortlessly. He expects his people to have permanent practical and, above all, intellectual tasks to be fully utilized. On the other hand, he tries very hard to please the two-legged friends (will to please), which means that the Border Collie can sometimes reach his strength limits.

**The right nutrition for small bundles of energy**

The Border Collie can be counted as a medium-sized dog. Border Collie dogs are usually very active dogs and require a lot of energy. Nevertheless, care should be taken during growth that the energy content is matched to the puppy's activity and not above it. Excessive energy supply in the feed can cause puppies to reach their genetically determined final weight earlier than intended or even exceed them, even though the skeleton is not yet sufficiently stable. This can result in misalignment of the limbs. Border Collie puppies, therefore, need an adequate supply of minerals, especially calcium and phosphorus, trace elements and vitamins, as well as an energy intake that is adapted to the respective activity level.

Feeding puppy food recommendations are based on the puppy's current weight and the expected weight as an adult dog. The weight of the same-sex parent animal serves as a guide. Also, the puppy's degree of activity is included in the calculation of the amount of food.

Always in action - fit with the right diet.

The Border Collie is a spirited and extremely bright dog. Since it was bred to be a herding dog, it needs a lot of activity. If the Border Collie is kept as a family dog, utilization is essential, both physically and mentally. The demands on the feed differ depending on the use and activity of the Border Collie. However, different requirements arise not only through use and breed. Each dog has its own needs, including nutrition. A dog's nutritional needs vary based on size, weight, age, and activity level. When it comes to nutrition, one should also consider the more frequent diseases of the musculoskeletal system.

After the Border Collie is fully grown, the diet should be changed to a diet designed for adult dogs. For dogs as active as the Border Collie, the food may contain more carbohydrates from which they can draw energy. However, with calm dogs, you should pay attention to a moderate proportion of carbohydrates to avoid obesity. In addition to the feed's activity level and composition, the amount of feed is also decisive for the weight. The number of treats and rewards should be subtracted from the daily ration. Whether you choose a suitable wet or dry food or a combination of both when choosing a food is a matter of taste for the dog and the owner.

## A well-deserved retirement - nutrition for senior dogs

Even the fittest and most active dog gets older and therefore have different needs than young or adult dogs. The physical changes that age brings with it result in different demands on the nutrition of senior dogs. Even Border Collies become cozier and calmer; their energy requirements decrease due to the decreasing activity. As a result, the feed's energy supply should be reduced so that the senior does not become overweight. Since some older dogs have a reduced sense of smell and taste, particularly tasty food can be beneficial.

## Feeding amount of a border collie senior

As a reward between meals and for training, Doka's chicken breast in pieces is suitable. They are low in fat and the right size to feed them while exercising. The Dokas chicken breast in pieces is natural, sugar-free, and suitable as a mono protein snack for sensitive dogs.

**The Doberman's Diet**

What should I put attention on?

Strong and muscular with an elegant and proud posture: the Doberman is not called the "ideal image of a dog" for nothing. It can - depending on gender - reach between 63 and 72 cm in size and weigh around 32 to 45 kg in its maximum of around thirteen years. The Doberman's mostly black or brown hair is short, hard, and dense and has no undercoat. It has rust-red markings on the head, chest, and legs.

The relatively young Dobermann breed came from Germany and was first bred in the 1870s by Friedrich Louis Dobermann (1834-1894) in Apolda, Thuringia. It is the only German breed named after its first known breeder.

Since the namesake worked as a dog catcher and tax collector in two very unpopular professional groups, he was not particularly popular with his fellow men. For his protection, he wanted to breed a dog that was not only scared off strangers by its appearance but could actually stop or deter strangers in case of doubt by its properties. Thus, from crossbreeding dogs with a great protective instinct, a lot of courage, and a quick-tempered character, a preliminary mix of Rottweilers and German Shepherds emerged. The resulting breed is agile and persistent, has keen senses, a great protective instinct, and a keen sense of right and wrong. He should be taught to assess the latter correctly; otherwise, the Doberman will decide at his discretion, which can sometimes be the undesirable direction from a human point of view. Also, a Doberman already reacts to minor stimuli.

Due to the characteristics mentioned, Dobermans were not only used as police dogs at the beginning of the 20th century, which gave them the nickname "gendarme dog," but above all, as working dogs, hunting dogs, and guard dogs. Thanks to their friendly and affectionate character, they are also ideal as family dogs, as they are also kind and open-minded towards children.

Loyal companion from the start

The Doberman can be counted among the medium to large dogs. With puppies of larger breeds, it is important to ensure that the food's amount is appropriate. The genetically determined final weight of a dog can be reached earlier than intended due to an excessive supply of energy in the food or even be higher. However, the skeleton is not yet designed for it. This can lead to malpositions of the limbs. Doberman puppies, therefore, need an energy supply that is adapted to their energy consumption and a balanced proportion of minerals, especially calcium and phosphorus, as well as trace elements and vitamins to get a strong skeleton.

Feeding puppy food recommendations are based on the puppy's current weight and the expected weight as an adult dog. The weight of the same-sex parent can serve as a guide. The amount of food also depends on the puppy's level of activity.

Good food for real guys

Depending on the Doberman's activity and area of application, his needs and the demands on his food differ. When on duty as a guard or protection dog, the need for energy and food is rather high. But even as a family member, the Doberman needs activity and sufficient exercise, be it through various types of games or sports programs and extensive hikes. Through regular and extensive exercise, the Doberman is a calm and balanced dog that is not satisfied with doing anything after training. Such a power pack naturally needs to be properly fed. Not only activity and breed bring certain needs with them; each dog has different characteristics and, thus, individual nutrition requirements. The nutrient and energy needs of a dog vary according to size, weight, and activity.

After the Doberman Pinscher is fully grown, the diet should be changed to a diet designed for adult dogs. For inactive and sporty dogs, the food may contain more carbohydrates for energy production. In contrast, less active dogs should have a moderate amount of carbohydrates to not become overweight. In addition to the level of activity and composition of the feed, the amount of feed is, of course, also decisive for the weight. The giving of treats and rewards should be taken into account.

The number of treats should be deducted from the daily ration. Whether you choose a suitable wet or dry food or combine both types of food is a matter of taste for the dog and the owner.

Still fit in old age - with the right diet.

Like humans, dogs are getting old and have different needs than younger dogs. The physical changes in old age place different demands on the dog's diet. The activity in senior dogs decreases, and the energy requirement decreases. So you should reduce the energy supply in the feed so that the senior does not gain weight. Since some older dogs have a reduced sense of smell and taste, particularly tasty food can be advantageous.

**The Golden Retriever's Diet**

What should I put attention on?

The Golden Retriever is one of the balanced and adaptable dog breeds. He was bred to be a hunting companion who was used together with other dogs. This explains its extraordinary compatibility with conspecifics, other animals, and also humans. Its will characterizes the Golden Retriever to obedience ("will to please") with a high level of attention and easy handling. This tendency makes him the perfect family dog who is very affectionate and gentle and prefers to participate in all family activities. Here he fits easily into his intended role. In addition to his poise, he is a happy and lively dog with a high urge to move, which is playful into old age.

All retriever breeds are known to originate from Newfoundland. In the 19th century, there was a brisk fish trade between England and Newfoundland. During their stay in Newfoundland, the English sailors watched the robust and weatherproof dogs on the island at work. They were thrilled that the water-loving dogs fetched boat lines out of the water and fish that had fallen out of the nets even in rough weather. The sailors brought some of these "little Newfoundlands" or "St. John's dogs "with them to England, where they were crossed with English hunting dogs. This resulted in the so-called "Wavy-Coated Retriever." In 1864 Lord Tweedmouth bought a similar Wavy-Coated Retriever with a fancy yellow color called "Nous." He mated the male with a Tweed Water female named "Belle." This breed was also known as persistent and good retrieval dogs. In the following 20 years, the offspring of "Nous" and "Belle" was mated with Wavy-Coated Retrievers and Tweed-Water dogs and crossed with Irish setters, the Golden Retriever. This was consequently used for hunting. It is mainly used for duck hunting to retrieve shot birds, also from the water. His intelligence and adaptability also qualify him as a guide, rescue, explosives, or drug search dog. This was consequently used for hunting. It is mainly used for duck hunting to retrieve shot birds, also from the water. His intelligence and adaptability also qualify him as a guide, rescue, explosives, or drug search dog. This was consequently used for hunting. It is mainly used for duck hunting to retrieve shot birds, also from the water. His intelligence and adaptability also qualify him as a guide, rescue, explosives, or drug search dog.

Strong bones and optimal growth through a healthy diet

The Goldie can be counted among the large dogs. Puppies of these breeds should not be fed too high energy levels to prevent them from growing too quickly. As a result of an excessive supply of energy in the feed, the genetically determined final weight can be reached earlier than intended and even be higher. However, the skeleton is not yet sufficiently stable. This can lead to malpositions of the limbs. Therefore, Golden Retriever puppies need adequate energy intake and a balanced intake of minerals, especially calcium and phosphorus.

For the Goldie puppy's healthy growth, you should pay attention to a needs-based and balanced proportion of energy, minerals, trace elements, and vitamins.

Feeding puppy food recommendations are based on the puppy's current weight and the expected weight as an adult dog. Here you can take the weight of the same-sex parent animal as a guide. Besides, the amount of food depends on the puppy's level of activity.

Whether at work or in the family - nutrition is what counts

The golden retriever is a versatile dog. It is ideally suited as a working and companion dog as well as a family dog, and it is also used as a retrieval, guide, detection, or rescue dog. The demands on the feed differ depending on the application. However, it is not just used and breeds that bring certain requirements with them; each dog also has different characteristics and individual nutritional requirements. A dog's nutritional needs vary based on size, weight, and activity. When it comes to nutrition, one should also consider the more common diseases of the Golden Retriever, such as allergies, obesity, and joint problems.

After the Goldie is fully grown, the diet should be switched to an adult dog diet. For active dogs, the food may contain more carbohydrates for energy production. In contrast, calm dogs should have a moderate carbohydrate content so that they do not become overweight. The fat content should also be in the medium range. In addition to the level of activity and composition of the feed, the amount fed is also decisive for weight. The giving of treats and rewards should be taken into account. The number of treats should be deducted from the daily ration. Whether you choose a suitable wet or dry food when choosing a food decides or combines both types of food is a matter of taste for the dog and the owner.

**Benefits of wet food**

The dog already absorbs liquid with the food, as wet food contains approx. 70% moisture

Wet food is usually tastier than dry food.

The amount of feed is greater due to the moisture content.

Wet food has a lower energy content than dry food, which can be particularly beneficial for dogs that tend to be overweight.

It has a long shelf life and is heated without preservatives.

Benefits of dry food

Dry food is usually cheaper than wet food.

Easy to portion and store, also suitable for on the go and when traveling

Good energy supply for active dogs

Loops can be counteracted by using large croquettes.

Lower packaging quantities than wet food

The bigger, the bigger

Dogs are also getting on in years. Older dogs have different needs than younger dogs. The physical changes make other demands on the diet—the physical changes associated with age place different demands on senior dogs' nutrition. As elderly dogs become less active, their energy needs to decrease. So you should reduce the energy supply in the feed so that the senior does not gain weight. Since some older dogs have a reduced sense of smell and taste, particularly tasty food can be advantageous.

**The diet of the Labrador Retriever**

Labrador feeding recommendation

Feeding a Labrador properly would not be an issue if the Labrador were allowed to decide - the main thing is that there is a large amount of food. Because this is one of those races that are not exactly picky about their food. Also, it is very difficult for us humans to resist the loyal and hungry looking dog eyes. These circumstances make it all the more difficult not to overfeed a Labrador.

The Labrador Retriever was originally used as a retriever when hunting. He is now considered the ideal family dog because he has a good-natured and friendly nature and likes to be around people. How active a Labrador is should guide its diet.

Healthy nutrition for a strong skeleton

Since the Labrador is a large dog, it is important that puppies of this breed are not fed too high energy levels so that they do not grow too quickly. The consequences of an over-supply of energy are a heavier weight than intended and the development of unstable bones. As a result, they cannot withstand the muscles' pull and the pressure caused by a higher weight, which can lead to malpositions of the limbs. Nevertheless, Labrador puppies need a lot of nutrients for optimal growth, as they can reach a weight of up to 35kg in a relatively short time.

For the Labrador puppy to have an ideal start to a healthy dog life, one should ensure that they have a balanced proportion of energy, minerals, trace elements, and vitamins appropriate to their needs.

Feeding puppy food recommendations are based on the puppy's current weight and the expected weight as an adult dog. Here you can take the weight of the same-sex parent animal as a guide. Also, the amount of food depends on the puppy's level of activity.

Out of its infancy - feeding the adult labrador.

When the Labrador is fully grown, the diet should be changed to food for adult dogs. In the case of a very active dog, the food can contain a few more carbohydrates for energy production. In contrast, a calm dog should ensure that the carbohydrate content is moderate to not become overweight. The fat content should also be in the medium range. Of course, the level of activity and the type of feed and the amount fed are decisive for the weight. The gift of treats and rewards should be taken into account here. The amount of treats is best deducted from the daily ration. Labrador Retrievers are more likely to struggle with joint problems, so foods are particularly suitable, containing components that support the joints, such as green-lipped mussels. Also, fibers such as carrots or apple pomace in the feed are beneficial for the intestinal flora.

Benefits of wet food:

The dog already absorbs liquid with the food, as wet food contains approx. 70% moisture

It is usually tastier than dry food.

Due to the moisture content, the amount of food is larger, which can be an advantage for the Labrador.

It has a lower energy content than dry food, which can be particularly beneficial for dogs prone to obesity.

It has a long shelf life and is heated without preservatives.

Benefits of dry food

It is usually cheaper than wet food.

Easy to portion and store, also suitable for on the go and when traveling

Good energy supply for active dogs

Loops can be contained with large croquettes.

Lower packaging quantities than wet food

It mostly already contains additives for the joints and other ingredients that can be beneficial for health.

## The golden autumn in dog life

The physical changes associated with age place different demands on the nutrition of senior dogs. The reduced movement reduces the energy requirement. So you should lower the energy supply in the feed so that the senior does not gain weight. Since some older dogs have a reduced sense of smell and taste, particularly tasty food can be advantageous.

## The diet of the pug

"A life without a pug is possible, but pointless." This saying comes from Loriot, one of the most famous pug admirers. Loriot was a fan of this breed, stars like Jessica Alba or Mesut Özil also fell for the pug. The pug can also become a celebrity himself, as in Sir Henry, the pug of society lady Uschi Ackermann, with his own Facebook page and pug collection. "You don't own a pug , you fall for it" is Uschi Ackermann's motto.

Anyone who knows a pug can easily understand this statement. The charming dog with the often grumpy or melancholy facial expression wins hearts by storm with his cheerful, humorous, and lively manner. He is neither aggressive nor quarrelsome towards other pets or other pets but is social and gets along well with everyone. However, consistent training is necessary, as the pug is very intelligent and has a feel for its owner's severity. It is adaptable and uncomplicated and, therefore, the ideal companion or family dog.

The breed history of the pug is not exactly clear; it probably comes from East Asia, most likely from China. It was a tradition there to breed small dogs with short, broad, and flatheads in common. The pug arrived in Holland as the first European country, probably by sea around 1600. William III. von Orange took a large number of Pugs with him to England to ascend the throne in 1688.

The House of Orange had a special relationship with this breed after a pug named Pompey had warned his master, Wilhelm the Silent, by barking loudly about an assassin and thus saved his life. In the 18th century, the pug experienced a boom, which is reflected in paintings, china, songs, and stories. He was mentioned in Wilhelm Busch and Johann Wolfgang von Goethe's works and, of course, in Loriot. The pug is one of the absolute fashion breeds, the trend towards breeding the "retromops" with changed properties such as long nose and neck is an important way in the right direction.

## The foundation for a healthy life - the right diet right from the start

The pug is one of the small dog breeds and reaches an ideal weight of approx. 6.3 to 8.1 kg with a height of approx. 26 to 34 cm. Since the pug belongs to the so-called brachycephalic breeds and has to struggle with breathing problems due to the round head shape with a short nose, additional excess weight should be avoided. You should pay attention to an appropriate amount of energy in the food. Otherwise, the pug will reach a higher weight than intended, and an unstable bone structure can develop.

The pug naturally has a compact build with good and firm muscles. Therefore, the pug needs sufficient exercise and a balanced, needs-based diet. This compactness can easily turn into obesity through improper nutrition in puppyhood. You should also keep an eye on the amount of food, as a pug won't stop eating on its own as long as there is still food in the bowl.

So that the little pug can start his life healthily, you should pay attention to a needs-based and balanced proportion of energy, minerals, trace elements, and vitamins in puppy food.

Feeding puppy food recommendations are based on the puppy's current weight and the expected weight as an adult dog. The weight of the same-sex parent animal is the guideline for this. The amount of food also varies with the puppy's activity level.

## Happy as the pug in the oat straw - feeding the adult pug

The adult pug should be fed a small adult dog food. Pugs are very attentive and sensitive to their people and adapt well to life situations and habits. Perhaps due to this property, there is the prejudice that the pug is lazy and, therefore, fat. An earlier breeding selection to the good eater is still noticeable in many pugs today. Therefore, as a pug owner, one should accommodate the temperamental, energetic dog and not slow it down.

This also makes it easier to avoid the risk of being overweight. However, in hot temperatures, you should pay attention to reduced exercise and use the early morning or late evening hours for a walk. The pug is more sensitive to high temperatures due to its anatomy with a short snout and the rudimentary turbinates associated with it.

Healthy snacks or croquettes from dry food can be used as treats for the pug. The number of treats should always be subtracted from the daily ration of the feed. Both wet and dry food is suitable for pugs. Here you can adjust to the dog's preference, or you can even feed both. The energy content (calories) in wet food is lower than in dry food. This can be especially beneficial for dogs that are prone to obesity.

The pug in his prime

Physical changes with age also change the demands on the diet and food of dogs. Reduced activity and movement reduce the energy requirement. So that the oldie does not gain weight, the energy content of the feed should be reduced. Nevertheless, nutritional requirements should be covered. The feed should also be of high protein quality. Since some older dogs have a reduced sense of smell and taste, particularly tasty food is advantageous.

## The diet of the Rhodesian Ridgeback

The Rhodesian Ridgeback - the only breed of dog in southern Africa - is strongly adapted to its original environment. You can tell at first glance that the Ridgeback was bred for lion hunting. With a large stature, an athletic, muscular build, and a thin, smooth coat, he has the ideal prerequisites for hunting in hot climates. His ancestors are the breeds of the colonial rulers from Great Britain and the Netherlands at that time, and there were probably also influences of the "Hottentot dog."

The Rhodesian Ridgeback is a loyal, loving family dog with a protective instinct who needs plenty of exercises to be happy and balanced. Also, the dogs are characterized by intelligence, strength of character, and courage, whereby they show little or no aggressiveness. Like all hunting dogs, the Rhodesians need experienced, sensible dog people familiar with species-appropriate training. As a sporty, activity-loving dog breed with a lot of stamina, the Ridgebacks like agility, obstacle sports, and exercises from hunting dog training. They are also excellent hunting dogs and, thanks to their talent for tracking, excellent rescue, or search dogs.

The agile, strong physique of the dogs is rounded off by high mobility. The fur is light brown and short. The alert, the attentive face, is framed by fine, triangular, floppy ears. Males reach a height of 63 to 69 cm with a weight of around 38 kilograms, bitches 61 to 66 cm in height, and around 32 kilograms. Breeders attach great importance to the back crest ("Ridge," or "Ridgeback"), which gave the dog breed its name. The comb is made of fur that grows against the direction of growth and comes in different shapes. It should be an average of 5 cm wide and develop hair swirls in specially specified arrangements. The back ridge carries risks for the development of a dermal sinus, a skin abnormality that extends deep into the tissue and, in turn, can sometimes promote infectious skin diseases.

The Rhodesian Ridgeback is on the list of dangerous dog breeds in Glarus's canton in Switzerland, and an application must be made there. In Bavaria, such an entry in a breed list was revoked in 2002 because it could not be proven that the breed animals are dangerous.

## Healthy nutrition in puppyhood - setting the course for a long dog life

The athletic ridge is counted among the large dogs. Puppies of these breeds should be given a diet with a moderate energy content tailored to their individual needs to not grow too quickly. The dog's genetically determined final weight can be reached earlier than intended due to an excessive supply of energy in the food and even be higher. However, the skeleton is not yet sufficiently stable.

This can lead to malpositions of the limbs. Therefore, rhodesian Ridgeback puppies need adequate energy intake and a balanced and needs-based intake of trace elements, vitamins, and minerals, especially calcium and phosphorus, for healthy growth.

Feeding puppy food recommendations are based on the puppy's current weight and the expected weight as an adult dog. The weight of the same-sex parent animal is suitable as a guideline. Besides, you adjust the amount of food to the activity level of the puppy.

Lion hunter or family dog - the main thing is that the diet is right.

The Rhodesian Ridgeback is a demanding dog that belongs in competent hands. The pronounced territorial behavior and the willingness to defend can only be handled through education and plenty of exercises. The teenage phase of this breed and thus the years of apprenticeship last longer than other dogs. Thanks to their prerequisites, Ridges belong to those dog breeds suitable as a guard, protection, rescue, and tracking dogs, which meets their need for movement. The Rhodesian Ridgeback also wants to be used to the full as a family dog, with dog sports such as obedience or agility and intelligence games, fetching, and much more. The demands on the food depend on the use of the dog. However, it is not just used and breeds with certain requirements; each dog also has different characteristics and, thus, individual nutritional requirements. A dog's nutritional needs vary based on size, weight, and activity. When it comes to diet, you should also consider the more common diseases of the Rhodesian Ridgeback, such as elbow and hip dysplasia and wobbler syndrome.

After the Ridgeback is fully grown, the dog's diet should be switched to adult food. For active dogs, the food may contain more carbohydrates for energy production. In contrast, calm and less active dogs should have a moderate carbohydrate content to not become overweight. The fat content should also be in the medium range. In addition to the level of activity and composition of the feed, the amount fed is also decisive for weight. The giving of treats and rewards should be taken into account. The number of treats should be deducted from the daily ration. Whether you choose a suitable wet or dry food when choosing a food decides or combines both types of food is a matter of taste for the dog and the owner.

Age does not protect against stupidity.

So that old dogs can still feel like young ones, it is advisable to adapt the food to the body's changes. Older dogs have different needs than younger dogs. The physical change creates different demands on the diet. The activity of senior dogs decreases; the energy requirement decreases. Consequently, one should reduce the feed's energy supply so that the senior does not gain weight. Since smell and taste are diminished in some older dogs, particularly tasty food has proven itself.

**The diet of the Rottweiler**

As one of the oldest dog breeds in Germany and the world, the Rottweiler belongs to the companion, service, and family dogs. Thanks to his self-confident, nervous, and attentive nature, it was already apparent at the beginning of the 20th century that he was ideally suited as a police dog, where he is still used today. One often hears about the - wrongly - bad reputation of the dog breed.

This is due to his strong drive to protect his family and, at the same time, a lot of strength that can lead to man-made problems in the wrong hands. With a good and early training already in the puppy age and similar socialization, the Rottweiler is characterized by human focus and good-naturedness and is therefore also suitable as a playmate for children. He is very affectionate, family-oriented, and adaptable.

Due to its high weight due to its strength, it is important to keep a Rottweiler in gentle but constant movement training from a young age. This ensures that the musculoskeletal system develops according to the body mass, and the animal remains fit. The Rottweiler then likes to use his power in dog sports and also develops a certain degree of joy in running.

Already in Roman times around 2000 years ago, the Rottweiler was used in a variety of ways: The ancient forerunner of the breed not only protected its people, for example, by accompanying the Roman legions across the Alps as an attentive working dog but also drove and tended cattle. Since the cattle drive was one of the butchers and cattle dealers' tasks, whose stronghold was Rottweil in the Middle Ages, the dog got the name "Rottweiler Metzgerhund," which is still used today.

The said butchers already used strong, strong dogs so that the Rottweiler can still reach a height at the withers of 56 to 68 cm and 42 to 50 kg. With this stature, you can deduce not only strength, but also mobility and endurance. The short, black fur with reddish-brown and delineated markings is distinctive for the dog breed. On the other hand, a long and relatively broad head with triangular ears and faithful, expressive eyes.

Getting up with the right paw - right from the start

The Rotti can be counted among the large dogs or Molossians. With Rottweiler puppies, it is essential to ensure that the amount of energy in the food is adjusted to not grow too quickly. As a result of an oversupply of energy in the food, the dog's genetically determined final weight can be reached earlier than intended and even higher. However, the skeleton is not yet sufficiently stable. This can lead to malpositions of the limbs. Rottweiler puppies, therefore, need an adequate energy intake and a balanced supply of minerals, especially calcium and phosphorus, to achieve a strong skeleton.

For a Rotti puppy's healthy growth, you should pay attention to a needs-based and balanced proportion of energy, minerals, trace elements, and vitamins.

A real guy needs real food.

Depending on the Rottweiler's activity and area of application, his needs and the demands on his feed differ. As a police or military service dog, the need for energy and food is high. However, even as a family dog, the Rotti loves to be exhausted by playing and romping or through sports programs and extensive hikes. With regular and extensive fitness training, the Rottweiler is a calm and relaxed dog who can also let all four be straight. Such a powerhouse naturally wants to be fed. However, it is not just used and breed that have certain needs. Each dog has different characteristics and thus, individual requirements for nutrition. The nutrient and energy needs of a dog vary according to size, weight, and activity. When it comes to nutrition, the Rottweiler's more common diseases, such as obesity and joint problems, should be taken into account.

After the Rottweiler is fully grown, their diet should be changed to a diet designed for adult dogs. In sporty and active dogs, the food may contain more carbohydrates for energy production. In contrast, calm and comfortable dogs should have a moderate carbohydrate content to not become overweight. The fat content should also be in the medium range. In addition to the level of activity and composition of the feed, the amount of feed is, of course, also decisive for the weight. The giving of treats and rewards should definitely be taken into account. The number of treats should be deducted from the daily ration. Whether you choose a suitable wet or dry food when choosing a food decides or combines both types of food is a matter of taste for the dog and the owner.

## Because of old iron - healthy old age with the right diet

Dogs are also getting on in years. Older dogs have different needs than younger dogs. The physical changes make other demands on the diet—the physical changes associated with age place different demands on senior dogs' nutrition. As elderly dogs become less active, their energy needs to decrease. So you should reduce the energy supply in the feed so that the senior does not gain weight. Since some older dogs have a reduced sense of smell and taste, particularly tasty food can be advantageous.

**The diet of the Shih Tzu**

Despite its name "lion dog," the Shih Tzu is neither dangerous nor scary. Only its appearance is reminiscent of its name. The Shih Tzu is rather known for his loyalty to the man and his family. He is happy, charming, and lovable likes to play with other conspecifics and children.

The small dog with a big heart is the ideal companion and needs a lot of attention but doesn't want to be alone. He is very robust and adaptable and likes to accompany his family on excursions. Due to its short snout, the Shih Tzu is not the right partner for long walks; it also likes to stay at home on the couch. He is considered loyal and docile, but he has his mind and can be very stubborn. A high degree of empathy is, therefore required for the education of Shih Tzu.

According to tradition, the breed originally came from Tibet and is one of the oldest dog breeds. The Shih Tzu is said to have lived in Tibet's monasteries as early as the seventh century.

According to stories, Buddha had a dog that turned into a lion. Hence the Chinese name Shih Tzu, which means "lion." The long fur is said to give the dog a lion-like appearance. From Tibet, the dog was brought to China as a tribute to the imperial court. Here the Shih Tzu enjoyed great popularity as a favorite in the palace. In the 20th century, the Shih Tzu made its way to Europe (Great Britain) and the USA, where it was recognized as a breed.

## Healthy diet - a cornerstone of a healthy dog life

The Shih Tzu is one of the small dog breeds and, depending on body size, can weigh between 4.5 and 7.5 kg. His posture is said to be arrogant. He is up to 27 cm high; a particular tendency to overweight is not known in the Shih Tzu. Nevertheless, concerning breathing difficulties due to their short muzzle, one should pay attention to the dog's weight. According to the breed standard, the Shih Tzu is an overly hairy dog with a thick undercoat. If not trimmed, the fur reaches a considerable length and falls like a flowing robe to the ground. As a puppy, you should spend a lot of time on grooming, and the puppy can get used to the necessary combing.

In addition to care and care, a needs-based diet is one of the cornerstones for a good start to a healthy dog life. Here you should pay attention to a needs-based and balanced proportion of energy, minerals, trace elements, and vitamins in puppy food.

Feeding puppy food recommendations are based on the puppy's current weight and the expected weight as an adult dog. The weight of same-sex parent can be used as a guide. Also, the amount of food depends on the puppy's level of activity.

Hatched from the nest and fully grown - feeding the adult Shih Tzu

When the Shih Tzu is fully grown, its diet should be switched to adult dog food. Although there is no known tendency towards obesity in the Shih Tzu, it doesn't hurt to keep an eye on the weight of your favorite. The long fur and short snout ensure that warmer temperatures are unfavorable for him and should therefore be avoided. High body weight could exacerbate this problem. The Shih Tzu is not known to be particularly fussy or sensitive to its food. Whether you give your Shih Tzu wet food or dry food feeds or mixes, both types of feed are up to you. Often, however, the dog decides based on its preferences. As a reward or for training, croquettes from the dry food or various small snacks are suitable. The amount of treats is best subtracted from the daily ration of the feed. When it comes to dry food, we recommend small croquettes adapted to the teeth of small dogs. Wet food is often popular because it is tastier than dry food. The liquid absorption is also higher with wet food since the moisture content is usually over 70%.

## Nutrition for the "best ager" of the Shih Tzu breed

An older, small dog needs a diet appropriate for its age and size, as the aging process causes physical changes—metabolism and activity decrease. An appropriately adapted diet with high acceptance and palatability can support the well-being of an older dog. He stays in shape for as long as possible, his food should be adapted to the specific signs of age and thus optimally promote healthy aging.

**The diet of the Weimaraner**

What should I put attention on?

As the oldest German pointing dog breed, the Weimaraner has been purely bred since around 1890 and has no crossings with other dog breeds. There are many theories about how the breed originated. Most likely, however, it seems that the Weimaraner was already held at the Weimar court by Grand Duke Karl August of Saxe-Weimar-Eisenach at the beginning of the 19th century. The breed was mainly bred for performance by foresters and professional hunters in central Germany.

With its height at the withers of 57 to 70 cm, the Weimaraner is one medium to large hunting dogs. With his sinewy build and strong muscles, he is an appropriate type of work. The females weigh about 25 to 35 kilograms, the males 30 to 40. The outer hair, which falls either short and smooth or soft and long, is usually silver, deer to mouse gray. The head and ears are usually lighter or have white markings. As a hunting dog with a persistent search, a love of challenges, and a strong motivation to complete tasks, he enjoys a special position among the pointing dogs. The Weimaraner shows its specialty in work after the shot by tracking down a game that has been shot or lost.

The versatile and reliable Weimaraner is not only good to use as a hunting dog but is also suitable as a very good protection and watchdog and, therefore, also as a family dog due to its pronounced territorial behavior and its watchful and non-aggressive nature. However, he needs a loving upbringing and a correspondingly careful, laborious, and consistent handling. With good and competent training, the Weimaraner can and wants to build a very solid bond with its owner. Although animals of the breed are sovereign, self-confident, and intelligent dogs, their hunting passion must be gently steered in the right direction in connection with their urge to move if they are not used as a hunting dog.

Setting the course for healthy growth: the right nutrition for puppies.

The Weimaraner is one of the large breeds of dogs. During growth, especially in puppies of larger breeds, it is necessary to feed them food with an appropriate amount of energy, as an excessive supply of energy can cause malpositions of the musculoskeletal system. In this case, a dog may reach its genetically determined final weight earlier than intended or possibly weigh even more, even though its skeleton is not stable enough to do so. To get strong bones and joints, Weimaraner puppies should be given food that meets their needs. Minerals, especially calcium and phosphorus, trace elements and vitamins and energy should be contained in the feed in the right amount.

To determine the feeding amount for a puppy, one orientates oneself on the dog's current weight and the assumed weight as an adult dog. It is believed that a puppy will reach a weight similar to that of its same-sex parent. Also, how active the puppy is is taken into account when determining the amount of food.

Proper nutrition for the aristocrat among dogs

The Weimaraner can show its abilities, talents, and merits in completely different areas of application. As a hunting dog, his original calling, as a protection and guard dog and as a family dog, he is versatile. Since the Weimaraner as a hunting dog has a strong need for exercise, this should be satisfied. However, a

Weimaraner that is used for hunting needs a higher supply of energy than a family dog. However, special needs arise from their activity and breed and each dog's characteristics. Dogs' nutritional and energy requirements differ based on size, age, weight, and activity level.

The Weimaraner should be given adult dog food after it is fully grown. Since this breed is one of the most active and active dogs, a food with a higher carbohydrate content is recommended. If your Weimaraner is one of the more comfortable specimens, a lower proportion of carbohydrates is an advantage, as otherwise, it could easily become overweight. Of course, the composition of the food and the level of activity are responsible for a dog's weight and the amount of food. The amount of rewards and treats that a dog receives on the side is also important. The number of treats should be deducted from the daily ration of food.

In the prime of life - the Weimaraner senior's diet. Dogs' needs for food change throughout their lives. Physical changes do not stop at senior dogs, either. The metabolism changes, the energy requirement decreases because the oldies are less active. To cater to dogs' age in terms of nutrition, it is advisable to switch to a senior food. Here the energy supply is reduced so that the senior does not gain weight. Some older dogs have a reduced sense of smell and taste, so a particularly tasty food can be beneficial.

# CHAPTER 5: LET'S MAKE DOG FOOD – DOG RECIPES

## PEANUT BUTTER COOKIES

Dogs love peanut butter, and these cookies are a great way to sneak some fish oil into your dog's diet. Fish oil improves your dog's coat, making it shiny, soft, and healthier.

Look for organic peanut butter in your grocery store. Many commercial brands of peanut butter have unhealthy hydrogenated oils and additives. Better yet, make your peanut butter with raw peanuts and peanut oil and process the mixture in your food processor.

### Ingredients

- 2 cups of flour (white or wheat if your puppy doesn't have wheat allergies)
- 1 cup of oatmeal
- 1/3 cup smooth peanut butter
- One tablespoon of honey

- 1/2 tablespoon of fish oil
- 1 1/2 cups of water

**Directions**

Preheat the oven to 350 degrees Fahrenheit.

Mix the flour and oats in a large mixing bowl. Pour a cup of water and stir until smooth. Add the honey, peanut butter, and fish oil and mix until all ingredients are well mixed.

Slowly add the water until the mixture is thick and pasty.

Lightly mix a cooking surface. Roll the dough onto the cooktop to make a 1/4 inch thick sheet.

Use a cookie cutter to create shapes. Place the cookies on a baking sheet and bake for 40 minutes.

Allow cooling completely before feeding.

**CHICKEN JERKY**

You can give these chicken jerky treats to your pup as an alternative to the raw hides bought in the store. The jerky is tough, so it will keep my dog busy for a while, and the chicken has a good amount of protein, which is good for a dog's muscle structure.

**Ingredients**

- 2 to 4 chicken breasts

**Directions**

Preheat the oven to 200 degrees Fahrenheit.

Remove excess fat from the chicken. Turn the chicken breast on its side and use a paring knife to cut the chicken breast into 1/8 inch strips.

Place the strips on a baking sheet—Bake for 2 hours.

Check the chicken before taking it out of the oven. It should be dry and hard, not soft or tough. Let the chicken cool completely before serving.

Store the jerky in an airtight container in the refrigerator for up to two weeks.

## FROZEN YOGURT POPS FOR DOGS

If your dog loves ice cubes in the kitchen, he will love these frozen treats. Made from human ingredients, they contain fruit juice and carrots that will give your pup an extra vitamin boost. Yogurt has calcium and protein and can help your dog digest food.

This recipe is for fat-free yogurt, which is a much healthier alternative to other types of yogurt, especially if your dog is overweight.

### Ingredients

- 6 ounces. A container of regular, non-fat frozen yogurt
- 1 cup of sugar with no added sugar
- 1/2 cup carrots, chopped

### Directions

Add the yogurt, fruit juice, and carrots to a medium bowl. Stir until ingredients are smooth and well blended.

Use a spoon to pour the mixture into the ice cube trays.

Freeze until ingredients are solid.

## FRUIT AND VEGETABLE STRIPS

These strips work as a cheaper alternative to the organic chewing products that are sold in pet stores. They also break apart easily, so you can serve smaller pieces as workout rewards. Fruits and vegetables are high in vitamin C, which can boost your dog's immune system.

### Ingredients

- One small sweet potato
- One medium banana
- One cup carrots, chopped
- 1/2 cup organic unsweetened applesauce
- Two cups of whole wheat flour (knows if your dog has allergies)
- 1/3 cup of water

- One cup of oatmeal

**Directions**

Cook the sweet potato in the microwave for eight to ten minutes, or until the inside is tender. Set aside and let cool.

Preheat the oven to 350 degrees Fahrenheit.

In a large mixing bowl, puree the banana and sweet potato using a hand pounder until smooth. Add the carrots, flour, and oats. Slowly add the applesauce and water as you mix.

The ingredients will form a soft batter. Roll the dough onto a lightly floured surface until the dough is 1/8 inch thick.

Cut the dough into strips.

Bake on a baking sheet for 25 minutes.

Store leftovers in the refrigerator for up to two weeks.

## BEEF AND VEGETABLE BALLS

Some dogs prefer meaty treats over sweet ones. These treats have a hearty, meaty flavor and aroma that all dogs love. When I did this, my dog

stood in front of the oven door, not waiting so patiently for the treats to cool down.

### Ingredients

- 2 6-ounce glasses of organic beef and vegetable baby food
- 1 cup whole wheat flour (or white substitute)
- 2 cups of dry milk
- 1 cup of water

### Directions

Preheat the oven to 350 degrees Fahrenheit.

Mix all the ingredients in a large mixing bowl.

Pour the mixture into large spoons on a baking sheet.

Bake for 12 to 15 minutes.

Let the treats cool completely—store leftover beef and vegetable balls in the refrigerator for up to five days.

## TURKEY AND VEGETABLE DINNER

This basic dog food recipe includes turkey for protein and vegetables for added vitamins and minerals. Turkey is lower in fat than beef, making it an ideal recipe for puppies, which might be shedding a few pounds.

### Ingredients

- 4 cups of water
- 1 pound of ground turkey
- 2 cups of brown rice
- 1 cup carrots, chopped
- 1 cup green beans, chopped
- One tablespoon fish oil (optional)

### Directions

Fry the ground turkey in a non-stick pan over medium heat until the meat is cooked through.

Put the turkey, brown rice, and water in a large saucepan and bring it to a boil.

Reduce the heat to medium-low and cook another 15 minutes, or until the rice is soft and tender.

Add the green beans and carrots and cook for another 5 to 10 minutes, until the vegetables are tender.

Let cool before serving.

Store extra dinners in the refrigerator for up to five days.

## CHICKEN CASSEROLE

This recipe uses chicken, a good source of protein, and lots of vegetables to create a flavorful mix. Green beans help your dog feel full, while vegetables promote a healthy intestinal tract.

### Ingredients

- Four chicken breasts
- 1/2 cup green beans, chopped
- 1/2 cup carrots, chopped

- 1/2 cup broccoli, chopped
- 1/2 cup of oatmeal.
- 4 cups low-salt chicken broth

Directions

Remove excess fat from the chicken breasts and cut the breasts into small nickel-sized chunks.

In a nonstick pan, cook the chicken breast over medium heat until it is no longer pink.

Add the chicken, vegetables, oatmeal, and chicken broth to a large saucepan and cook over medium heat until the carrots are tender - about 15 minutes.

Let cool before serving.

Store leftovers in the refrigerator for up to five days.

**PUPPY CHILI**

Dogs need large amounts of protein to keep them healthy and active. Your puppy should get most of its protein from whole meat sources, such as fresh chicken. Beans have a good amount of protein too.

This recipe mixes chicken, beans, and vegetables into a healthy and tasty mix.

**Ingredients**

- Four chicken breasts
- 1 cup kidney beans, drained
- 1 cup black beans, drained
- 1 cup of carrots, diced
- 1/2 cup tomato paste
- Four cups of chicken broth

**Directions**

Remove the excess fat and dice the chicken breast into pieces the size of a nickel.

In a pan over medium heat, cook the chicken breast over medium heat until it is no longer pink.

In a large saucepan, add the chicken, beans, carrots, tomato paste, and chicken broth and cook over medium heat until heated through - about ten minutes.

Let the mixture cool before serving.

Store chili in the refrigerator for up to five days.

Pro tip: you can add 1/2 tablespoon of fish oil to this recipe. The flavors are strong enough that even picky eaters won't notice the added healthy ingredient.

## BEEF RAGOUT

This dog-approved version of the beef stew contains meat for protein, vegetables for vitamins, and flavor sauce. This is a great alternative to wet commercial dog foods.

### Ingredients

- 1 pound of beef stew meat
- One small sweet potato
- 1/2 cup carrots, diced
- 1/2 cup of flour
- 1/2 cup green beans, diced
- 1/2 cup of water or organic vegetable oil, plus one tablespoon of vegetable oil for frying

### Directions

Cook the sweet potato in the microwave for 5 to 8 minutes until firm but tender. Put aside.

Cut the stew pieces into smaller pieces the size of a nickel.

Cook the stews in a tablespoon of vegetable oil over medium heat for 10-15 minutes, or until well done.

Remove the chunks of beef from the pan and reserve the pieces of dripping fat.

Dice the sweet potato.

Heat the drops over medium-low heat. Slowly add flour and water to the dripping water to make a thick sauce.

Add the sweet potato, carrots, meat ,and green beans into the sauce and stir to coat.

Cook until the carrots are tender - about ten minutes.

Serve cool.

Store the remaining stew in the refrigerator for up to five days.

Pro tip: you can buy pre-made sauce at some health food stores. This can save you time when preparing this food.

## FRUIT PARFAIT FOR DOGS

Your dog deserves a delicious dessert every now and then. This parfait mixes fruit and dairy, so it tastes great, but it also gives your pup a nice helping of vitamins and protein.

### Ingredients

- 1/2 cup of plain, fat-free yogurt
- 1/2 cup strawberries, diced
- 1/2 cup blueberries, diced
- 1/2 cup applesauce

### Directions

Put all ingredients in a medium bowl until the yogurt is smooth, and the fruits are well mixed.

Serve in small quantities.

Store in the refrigerator for up to seven days.

## DOG BISCUITS - basic recipe

### Ingredients

- 150g flour
- 50g oatmeal
- One tablespoon olive oil
- One egg

### Directions

You can add, for example, grated apple, carrot, beet, pumpkin, garlic, cheese, or spinach to this base.

Make a dough (add a little water as needed), roll out the pancake, place on a baking sheet, and bake at 180 degrees for about 30-35 minutes. After cooling, break it as needed.

## CRACK BISCUITS

### Ingredients

- Crackling biscuits for dogs
- 300g of oatmeal
- 200g greaves
- One egg
- Two cloves of garlic
- a little water

### Directions

You mix everything by hand together. It takes a moment of patience before the greaves loosen, then you make the patties and bake them at 175 ° C for about 30 minutes. The cookies smell beautiful; the combination of greaves and garlic is amazing. Keep the cookies in a box in the fridge, and I think they are even better after two days.

## MILLS WITH GOAT MILK

## Ingredients

- 250g millet
- 100g goat's milk powder (e.g., Dromes of goat's milk porridge )
- Two eggs
- Two tablespoons cannabis seeds
- Two tablespoons sunflower seeds
- Two tablespoons flaxseed
- One tablespoon germ oil

## Directions

Boil the millet until soft, mix the goat's milk with 400 ml of hot water to form a porridge. You then mix all the ingredients together. Place baking paper on a baking sheet and spread the millet on it in a thinner layer (as on a bun)—Bake at 180 ° C for about 40 minutes. After cooling, cut into smaller pieces and use either as a treat or as a side dish to raw meat or canned food. Store in the refrigerator for up to 14 days.

## LIVER BISCUITS

### Ingredients

- 150g flour
- 100g oatmeal
- 100g of boiled liver
- 30g grated cheese
- One clove of garlic
- One teaspoon oil

### Directions

Mix everything together, add water as needed so that the dough does not stick. Roll out the pancake, cut into pieces of any size, transfer to a baking sheet and bake at 180 ° C for about 30 minutes until the biscuits are slightly browned.

Instead of the liver, you can put boiled chicken breast or tuna from a can.

## MEAT PATTIES

Every dog will go crazy for meat patties. They are simple, and you supply him with the nutrients themselves.

**Ingredients**

- 250 g minced meat (ideally mixed pork and beef)
- egg
- mug of oatmeal
- little marjoram
- garlic clove (in small quantities once in a while it does not harm the dog)

**Directions**

Mix all the ingredients in the bowl into a solid mixture. Make thin patties and place them on a baking sheet. Bake for about twenty minutes at 175 ° C . You can finally break the patties into smaller pieces so that the dog can eat better.

## CARROT BISCUITS FOR DOG PUPAE

Support the dog peepholes, which are looking at you reproachfully, because the muzzle under them has not received any goodness for a long time. Bake the dog carrot biscuits so that his eyesight is like a perch!

## Ingredients

- egg
- Four tablespoons lukewarm water
- 200 g finely grated carrots
- 250 g wholemeal flour
- ½ baking powder
- Three tablespoons vegetable oil

## Directions

Beat the eggs with oil and then add the other ingredients. Roll out the mixture, and if the dough sticks to your hands, add a little more flour. Cut the biscuits with the cutters you have on hand and stack them on a baking sheet. Bake in a preheated oven at 175 ° C for about 15 minutes, following the biscuits' color – the finished ones are golden.

## CHEESE APPETIZERS FOR GOURMETS

If your pet is constantly drenched in a cheese of any kind, give him the joy of cheese cookies.

### Ingredients

- mug of grated cheese
- cup of flour
- a cup of milk
- spoons of butter

### Directions

Mix loose ingredients with butter and add milk. The result should be a non-stick dough. Roll out the pancake and cut out the pancakes that will fit the size of the hairy diner. Then bake on a baking paper sheet in the preheated oven for about 10 minutes at 175 ° C.

## APPLE COOKIES FOR FRUIT LOVERS

Can your dog also beat up apples? He is constantly begging for a piece of sweet fruit, so you don't have much leftover from the snack yourself? Make him happy with apple biscuits. You will see that he will thank you properly.

## Ingredients

- apple
- 150 g of flour
- ½ teaspoons of cinnamon
- 75 g of oatmeal
- One tablespoon sunflower oil
- 40 ml of water

## Directions

Peel an apple and grate it roughly. Mix loose ingredients in a bowl, add apple and oil. Combine everything into a non-sticky dough, which you then roll out and place completely on a baking sheet. Pierce it in several places with a fork and cut it into pieces of a size that will suit your dog—Bake in a preheated oven at 175 ° C for 30 minutes. After removing the oven, remove the result from the plate with the paper and let it cool down. Only then separate the pieces from each other.

## CHEESE BISCUITS

Ingredients:

- 1 cup wheat flour
- 1 cup grated cheese (ideally cheddar type)
- One tablespoon softened butter
- ½ cup milk

Procedure:

Mix flour and cheese, then add softened butter. Gradually add milk to the processed mass until you get a firm and non-sticky dough (you may not need the entire amount of milk, depending on the flour).

Roll out the dough into a thin roller and cut it into wheels (their size depends on the dog). Place it on a baking sheet lined with baking paper and bake for a few minutes at 180 degrees (you can tell that the biscuits are done by turning them pink). Allow them to cool and store in the refrigerator to keep them fresh for a long time.

## SPICY BISCUITS

**Ingredients:**

- ½ a cup of honey
- ¾ a cup of unsweetened apple juice
- ¼ a cup of molasses
- One egg
- Two and ¼ a cup of flour
- Two teaspoons baking powder
- One teaspoon ginger
- One teaspoon cinnamon
- ½ teaspoons ground cloves

Procedure:

Preheat the oven to 180 degrees. In a bowl, mix honey, apple juice, molasses, and eggs. Mix the flour, baking powder, and spices in the second bowl, then gradually incorporate the loose mixture into the prepared liquid mixture. Then shape the biscuits on a baking sheet covered with baking paper using a spoon (the dough is a bit thinner). Bake for about eight to ten minutes (depending on the size of the biscuits).

## SARDINE BISCUITS

Ingredients

- Two packs of sardines in their juice
- One tomato puree
- 500g oatmeal
- Two eggs
- baby semolina
- hemp flour
- poppy seed oil
- flax seeds
- water

Procedure

Put two packs of sardines in their juice, one tomato puree, 500g oatmeal (we can use mixed), two eggs, dust with baby semolina and hemp flour, pour poppy seed oil (excellent source of calcium), add light flaxseed, and as needed, we add water.

Mix into a thick mixture, which is then spread on a baking sheet lined with baking paper. Bake in a preheated oven to about 150 - 175 degrees for about 10-15 minutes.

After cooling, we cut and serve :-)

## SPINACH CRACKERS

### Ingredients

- One pack of spinach puree
- 500g oatmeal
- Two eggs
- baby semolina
- hemp flour
- a drop of olive oil
- water as needed

Procedure

We mix all the ingredients in a bowl and create a thick mass, spread on a baking sheet. Bake in the oven at 150 - 175 degrees for about 10 - 15 minutes.

Let cool and then slice. Store in the refrigerator, or we can freeze.

## TURKEY BISCUITS FOR SWEET TONGUES

If you want to make your sweet dog friends happy and you like to prepare food at home, there are wonderful baked turkey biscuits with cheese. They will take a maximum of an hour, and you will certainly not need dog assistants to watch the oven :

### Ingredients

- 1 ½ cup oatmeal
- 1 ½ cup brown rice flour
- ½ cup swiss cheese
- ½ cup minced turkey (pre-cooked and dried)
- ½ cup oat bran
- One tablespoon dried parsley
- One egg
- ½ cup of water

### Procedure

Preheat the oven to 175 degrees. Mix all the ingredients except the water, which we add gradually and mix until the dough is formed. It may not be necessary to add all the water; if the dough is too wet, we will add flour.

Roll out the dough and cut out the shapes with a rake or a cutter. Transfer to baking paper and bake in the oven for about 22-27 minutes or until the dough is golden brown. Allow to cool completely and store in a closed container in the refrigerator.

## BART'S TUNA BALLS

Christmas is approaching, and we can also prepare delicious cookies for the dogs. These beautiful fragrant balls are not only very popular but also easy to prepare ;-)

### Ingredients

- whole tuna in its juice
- a handful of wheat flour
- a handful of crushed flakes
- one yolk
- a little water to join the dough

### Procedure

Mix all the ingredients and roll out the balls—Bake in a preheated oven for 180 degrees for about 20 minutes.

We serve the dog chilled and stored it in a paper bag, which we leave half-open so that the biscuits harden nicely.

## TUNA CRACKERS

### Ingredients

- One can of crushed tuna in its juice
- One egg
- 2 cups finely ground oatmeal
- One carrot finely grated

### Procedures

Mix the ingredients and make a dough. If the dough is dry and cannot be combined, add a drop of water. We form small balls, which we spread into patties. Bake on a baking sheet on baking paper at 150 to 170 degrees C for about 15 to 20 minutes.

## TRIPE CROQUETTES

### Ingredients

- 500g wholemeal flour
- 250g beef tripe
- soup spoon of flax seeds
- One egg a
- pinch of dried garlic
- herbs, we can add according to your imagination - e.g., marjoram, chives.

### Procedure

Mix the beef tripe and add it to the flour. We season all the ingredients in a bowl and then roll them on a roll. The dough should not stick but be "just right" (if necessary, add more flour).

If you have a meat grinder with a candy attachment, shape the croquettes with a grinder. It's faster than rolling out dough and slicing. We put the pieces on a baking sheet with baking paper and put them in a heated oven. Bake until the croquettes have a golden, nice color.

If you want your mum to last for a while, bake slowly and dry more. To increase durability, leave them in the air for about three days to dry.

## BEEF STICKS

### Ingredients

- 500g wholemeal flour
- 200 - 250g beef
- Two eggs a
- pinch of dried garlic a pinch of
- baking powder
- One tablespoon olive oil
- water as needed

### Procedure

Pour wholemeal flour into a bowl, add ground beef, eggs, garlic, baking powder, oil, and, if necessary, water. We start making the dough with a wooden spoon, which we then roll out on a rolling pin. We will start making a firmer, non-sticky dough.

We can easily mix other flour.

After working out the dough, divide it into several parts and roll out pancakes about 3 mm thick and start cutting the sticks with a spade.

Put the sticks on a baking sheet—Bake in a preheated oven to a lower temperature, about 20 minutes. We dry rather than bake. After the stick has cooled down, transfer it to the tray. If you leave them at room temperature, where it is not humid, the biscuits will dry out more, and thus their shelf life will be extended for a very long time.

---

## OTHER ADDITIONAL RECIPES

Vegetable puree for the dog: 15 minutes

Dogs are animals that, like humans, can eat meat and vegetarian dishes. "A vegetarian diet does not have to cause a nutritional deficiency in a dog if it is balanced.", notes Donald R. Strombeck in his handbook.

An easy option is to cook mashed lentils, which can then be mixed with rice. If you need to soak the vegetables the night before soaking and use a quick container, the processing time will not exceed 15 minutes.

Strombeck recommends using tofu (soy milk curd, which contains high-quality protein) to prepare meatless meals if they intend to make these recipes part of the dog's usual diet. However, tofu can increase the price of food. And it is possible to do without vegetarian food being the only one that can be put in a can. In this case, vegetable dishes are usually cheaper for a handbag in addition to animal nutrition options.

## TUNA SNACK PER CAN: 12 MINUTES

Fast and tasty. The elaboration of these fish delicacies for the dog allows several possibilities. Perhaps the easiest - though quick - is to choose tuna whims.

The elaboration is as follows. The content of several cans of tuna is crushed (better, low salt content and without oil). Add beaten eggs and half a glass of hot water to prepare the dough. The mixture is moved using a fork. Once it has a homogeneous consistency, the whims are introduced into the oven (about ten minutes) or in the microwave, allow them to cool slightly, and voilà! They are ready to please a furry friend.

## SCRAMBLED EGGS WITH "SOMETHING": 9 MINUTES

Broken or fried eggs (with a little oil) and mixed in iron with "something," as suggested by dog feeding expert Carlos Gutiérrez in his blog Nutritional Expert, are a fast and economical meal will reward a dog.

Some green beans (cooked or leftovers), a little cooked pasta (same), or a few pieces of ham (no fat or bones) perfectly accompany this simple recipe for a dog that doesn't take more than nine minutes to prepare. It is only important not to add salt, especially if you add animal ingredients to eggs.

### Macaroni for the dog: 13 minutes

Simple pasta can become a nutritious and inexpensive home design for a can. The dough chosen should be short: macaroni or similar (and not elongated, spaghetti) so that it can be chewed without any problems. If the water is boiled in a particular heater (which speeds up cooking), the paste can be prepared in about 13 minutes.

Some broken or boiled eggs in the form of a tortilla (with a little oil) will be the perfect addition to these macaroons. Preparing the dish can be completed with a few chicken breasts and even a can of sardines, better if they are natural.

## RICE WITH VEGETABLES

Cereals and Vegetables are excellent homemade dog food. To prepare this nutritious and tasty recipe for rice with vegetables for your dog, you need to:

**Ingredients**

- 2 cups brown rice
- Sliced chicken or turkey meat
- Two carrots
- 1 cup broccoli
- 1 cup spinach
- Two potatoes
- 4 cups water or chicken broth

**Direction**

Wash all vegetables well and cut them into small pieces.

Boil water or broth and cook for 30-40 minutes until everything is soft.

On the other hand, cook rice.

Mix everything. If you wish, you can pass the vegetables through a shredder to make it even smaller or stretch it.

## TUNA ROULADE

Fish are also great natural food for our pets. However, try not to abuse bluefish in your diet; it is good for occasional consumption. You can vary with white fish such as hake.

To prepare this homemade tuna roll for dogs, you need:

### Ingredients

- One can of tuna in water.
- One teaspoon olive oil
- One branch of celery
- One large carrot
- One teaspoon lemon juice
- Four tablespoons cottage cheese

### Directions

Crush all ingredients until you get a formable paste.

Add lemon juice and mix well.

Make a croissant or sausage with it.

Prepared! Just cut down on portions as you need. Ah, Watch out for the cheese! It's good in small portions, but don't abuse it, or it might feel bad. When eating cheese, take good care of your dog. Some dogs are intolerant to lactose and can cause diarrhea.

## MEAT PIE

What would dogs be without meat! Meat is the basis of natural food for dogs and cannot be missing from the diet. They are carnivorous animals!

These are home-chopped ingredients for dogs:

### Ingredients

- 2 cups brown rice for dogs.

- 3 cups of water
- Two grated potatoes
- Four grated carrots
- Two chopped celery sticks
- 2.5 kg of sliced chicken
- Eight eggs
- Three tablespoons olive oil
- 1 cup oatmeal

**Directions**

Cook the rice and let it cool.

In a bowl, mix the vegetables and eggs and mix well.

Add olive oil, oatmeal, and rice.

Spread the mixture on a baking sheet and bake for 30-40 minutes at 200 ° C.

Let it cool, and you will be ready to cut into portions as you see fit.

**ICE CREAM FOR BANANA DOGS**

Finally, dessert, homemade ice cream for dogs.

## Ingredients

- Four natural yogurts
- Two tablespoons peanut butter
- Three ripe bananas, peeled and crushed.

## Directions

Stir all the ingredients until they are cleaned.

Fill the mixture into plastic cups.

Put the cups in the freezer until the mixture freezes.

Once you freeze, you can take it and send it to your dog.

The remaining cups of ice cream can be stored in the freezer for two weeks and gradually removed.

## Ten Cooking Tips For Your Dog

1. Home cooking is the possibility of feeding a dog. Still, it can replace commercial meals (feed and cans) only if a balanced diet is prepared under veterinarian or dog nutrition supervision.

2. Every dog has different nutritional needs, which depend not only on their weight. Therefore, it is not valid to get a home diet and recalculate the necessary amounts depending on the dog's kilograms.
3. Homemade meals allow this to be safely cooked for allergic dogs or with special nutritional requirements. But always with the consent of a veterinarian.
4. Most home recipes for a dog do not serve as an exclusive diet: in these cases, commercial nutritional supplements - especially vitamin B12 supplements in a vegetarian diet - are necessary and should be prescribed by a doctor.
5. High-end commercial diets are carefully prepared. Its nutrients and ingredients are balanced to meet the needs of dog food. To achieve this with the home diet, it must be carefully designed by a dog nutritionist.
6. Cooked food for dogs must not contain an excessive number of ingredients: the dog's digestive system is not the same as humans. Four or five is enough.
7. Dogs do not allow frequent changes in feeding as we receive humans. This explains the importance of developing a healthy and balanced diet with veterinary supervision.
8. To design a home diet for your dog, it is essential to know your dietary needs: the number of daily calories you need and the number of vitamins and other essential nutrients.
9. There are certain forbidden foods They are toxic for the dog, even in small amounts. His chocolate, onions, garlic, raisins, grapes, and avocados are among them. Salt and sugar should also not be avoided and bypassed raw pork.

10. Food allergies in dogs are not strange. When they are diagnosed, it is necessary to remove the components that make them. And to avoid dangers, it is necessary to gradually incorporate new components of the dog's home diet in small amounts.

# CONCLUSION

Cooking for a dog at home is possible, And in addition to controlling the components of your diet, you can save money. Preparing food doesn't have to be laborious or stealing too much time.

Whether you are a long-time or a freshly baked dog owner: the right dog nutrition plays a crucial role in life with a four-legged friend. It should too: after all, a dog's health is closely related to food. Physical well-being, vitality, and your four-legged friend's lifespan can be influenced and increased with the right food. On the other hand, the wrong food can make the dog sick. Obesity, diabetes, cardiovascular diseases, skeletal and joint diseases, Kidney disease, and even cancer can be triggered by poor diet. No wonder that the topic is so much in focus and that there are almost as many opinions on the right diet in specialist literature, guides, and internet forums as there are dog breeds.

But which of these is the perfect food for my dog? This question can not be answered, generally. After all, not all dogs are the same. Depending on size, age, state of health, weight, and activity level, the food demands are also very different. You can only find out the perfect food for your animal individually for yourself. Ultimately, it has to take into account not only your pet's needs but also your life situation. What is practicable for one person in everyday life means a great challenge for the other. Price, route of delivery, and time certainly play a role in deciding which feeding method is best. It is important that you can give the food that is good for your dog in the long term. Because a frequent change of feed is often very stressful for the animal organism, diarrhea, gas, and other digestive problems can result from too much change in the food bowl.

Unfortunately, the question of the perfect food for your dog cannot be answered here. However, below you will find the most important criteria to help you find the optimal dog food.

CPSIA information can be obtained
at www.ICGtesting.com
Printed in the USA
BVHW071934130421
604819BV00008BA/599

9 781802 662085